W0106349

Springer-Verlag Italia Srl.

Giovanni Broggi (Ed.)

Craniopharyngioma
Surgical Treatment

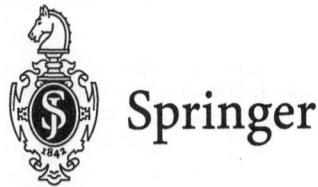 Springer

GIOVANNI BROGGI, M.D.
Istituto Nazionale Neurologico "C. Besta"
Via Celoria, 11
I - 20133 Milan

ISBN 978-3-540-75001-7   ISBN 978-88-470-2291-1 (eBook)
DOI 10.1007/978-88-470-2291-1

This work is subject to copyright. All rights are reserved, whether the whole or part of the material is concerned, specifically the rights of translation, reprinting, reuse of illustrations, recitation, broadcasting, reproduction on microfilm or in any other way, and storage in data banks. Duplications of this publication or parts thereof is permitted only under the provisions of the German Law of September 9, 1965, in its current version, and permission for use must always be obtained from Springer-Verlag. Violations are liable for prosecution under the German Copyright Law.

© Springer-Verlag Italia 1995
Originally published by Springer-Verlag Italia, Milano in 1995.

The use of general descriptive names, registered names, trademarks, etc. in this publication does not imply, even in the absence of a specific statement, that such names are exempt from the relevant protective laws and regulations and therefore free for general use.

Product liability: The publishers cannot guarantee the accuracy of any information about dosage and application contained in this book. In every individual case the user must check such information by consulting the relevant literature.

Foreword

The Paolo Zorzi Association for Neurosciences was founded in 1978 to promote scientific and clinical research in the field of neuroscience, with particular attention to neurooncology, epileptology, and those diseases that cause movement disorders in infancy and childhood.

During these past years the activity of the Association has increasingly developed, making important contributions to the study of these diseases and to their treatment by integrating the basic sciences and clinical research.

Within the Association, a Scientific Commitee formed by Giovanni Broggi, the promoter of the workshop whose proceedings are published in this book, Giuliano Avanzini, Lucia Angelini and Roberto Spreafico, who all work at the Istituto Nazionale Neurologico "C. Besta" in Milan, guarantees that the sponsored initiatives correspond to the goals of the Association.

The many papers published in reputable international journals and in books of great scientific relevance - the latest of which is this one - testify to the activity of the Association. Moreover, the Association directly supports some research programs by awarding grants to promising young neurologists in Italy and abroad and by promoting scientific congresses on neurosurgery, neuropsychiatry, neuroanatomy and neurophysiology. An example of this was the organization of the Workshop: "Craniopharyngioma: Surgical Treatment" held in Milano, Italy, in May 1993.

We thank Giovanni Broggi and all those who made this Workshop a success and the publication of this book possible, and the Association whishes to be able to promote congresses of the same scientific level in the near future.

Dr. Franco Santamato, President
Paolo Zorzi Association
for Neurosciences

Table of Contents

Neuropathology of Craniopharyngioma

A. Allegranza

Craniopharyngiomas are benign epithelial tumors of congenital malformative origin. They are thought to originate, though this is still under debate, from remnants of Rathke's pouch, which is a protrusion of the roof of the stomodeum or primitive oral cavity (Russell and Rubinstein 1977). These remnants, called Erdheim's remnants (hence the name Erdheim's tumor) are often found in the pituitary stalk, in the sellar, parasellar location or even in the sphenoid bone. Tachibana et al. (1994) have recently demonstrated by immunohistochemical study that in the cells of the adenohypophysis and in craniopharyngiomas glycoprotein P (PGP) present in the cytotrophoblast and human chorionic gonadotropin (HCG) are coexpressed. These data suggest that craniopharyngiomas produce HCG-like peptides; therefore they can be considered the only squamocellular tumors that, in the sellar region, originate from neuroendocrine precursors.

Craniopharyngiomas are usually located over the sellar diaphragm and less frequently in the sella. Their rupture in the third ventricle is very rare (Fig. 1). The sphenoid bone and exceptionally the paranasal sinuses, nasal pharynx, and the pineal region and the pontocerebellar angle have been reported as ectopic localizations.

Two types are classified: the classic type, called adamantinomatosus, and the papillary type (Burger and Vogel 1982). Transitional forms have also been described (Petito et al. 1976; Szeifert et al. 1993).

The *adamantinomatous craniopharyngioma* is found in young subjects during the first two decades. It is commonly found as a suprasellar lesion involving the pituitary stalk, chiasm, optic nerve, and contiguous vessels up to the ventricle (Figs. 2,3). Macroscopically, it has solid and cystic areas: the cavities of various sizes contain fluid material, sometimes dense, yellow, dark, similar to "motor oil." Histologically, in the solid areas, it is formed by clusters, cords, and sheets of epithelial cells that, at the periphery, are arranged like a palisade, while in the center, for a process of differentiation, they are loosely arranged and assume a starry form, creating patterns which

Consultant pathologist, Dept. of Neurosurgery, Istituto Nazionale Neurologico "C. Besta", Via Celoria 11, 20133 Milan, Italy

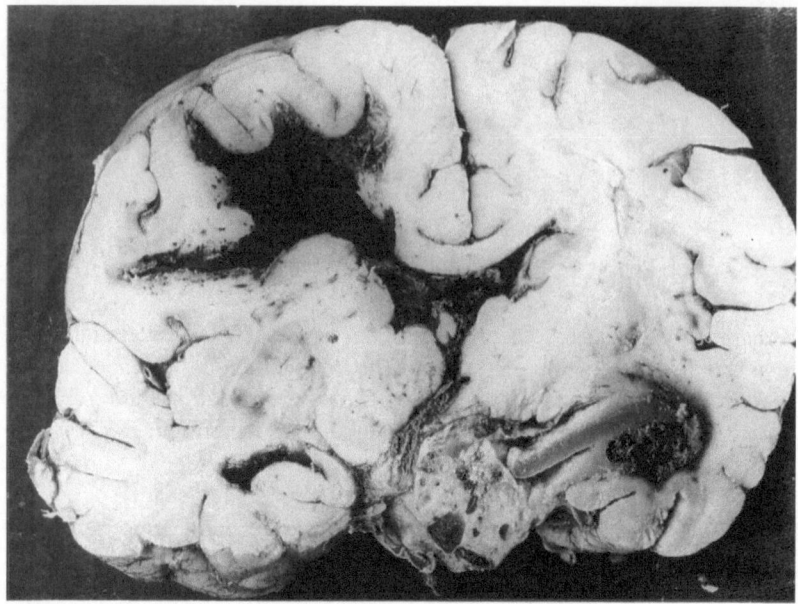

Fig.1. Craniopharyngioma located in the interpeduncular-chiasmatic fossa, spreading to the right sylvian fissure. In a frontal section, it shows a solid cystic hemorrhagic aspect. In the progression toward the third ventricle it caused a sudden and fatal hemorrhage of the white matter of the left hemisphere

are reminiscent of the "stellate reticulum" of the pulp of the enamel organ and of the mandibular adamantinomas (thus it is called adamantinomatous craniopharyngioma) (Fig. 4). Clusters of squamous epithelial cells, keratinized pearls, and calcifications are observed. No keratohyalin granules are present in the epithelial squamous elements.

In the cystic areas the cavities are filled with glycoproteic material mixed to cholesterol crystals, squamous dying cells, and cellular debris. This material can reach the adjacent stroma and cause formation of granulomas with foreign body giant cells surrounding negative images of cholesterol crystals.

Papillary craniopharyngioma is found mainly in adults. It is rarely suprasellar and more frequently it develops in the third ventricle. Macroscopically, it appears as a solid mass with small cavities well delimited and without the presence of "motor oil" fluid. Microscopically, it is formed by cords of well differentiated squamous epithelial cells that are sustained by fibrovascular septa, thus giving the aspect of papillary structures (Fig. 5). Adamantinoid aspects, keratinized whorls, calcifications, cholesterol deposit, and granulomatous reactions with giant cells are lacking.

Szeifert et al. (1991), on the basis of histochemical and ultrastructural studies, think that the elements that delimit the cavities of craniopharyngi-

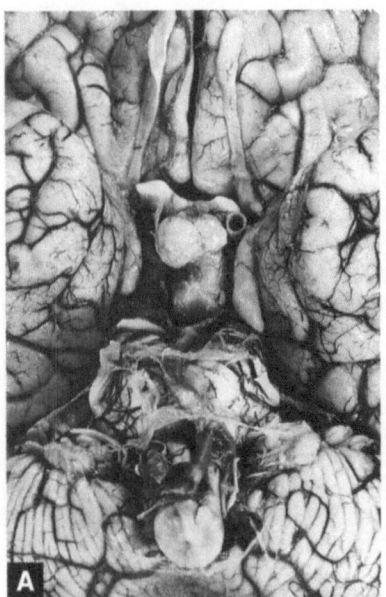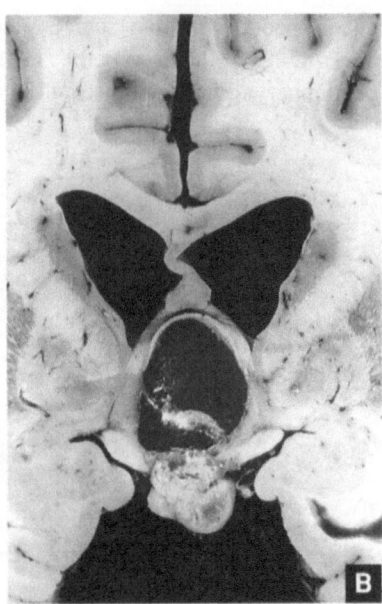

Fig. 2 A, B. Behind the optic chiasm (**A**) presence of a nodule, well delimited, that in a frontal section (**B**) is connected to a microcystic mass separating the optic tracts, raising the floor of the third ventricle, where it assumes the form of a wide cystic cavity occupied by homogeneous dark material. Female, 60 years old

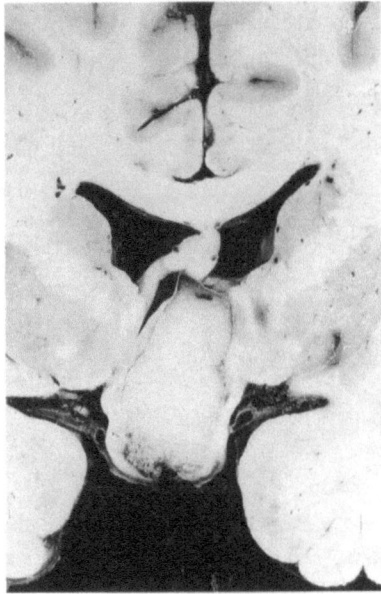

Fig. 3. Frontal section at the level of the basal nuclei. The lesion is mainly cystic and well delimited and appears to nest in the third ventricle. Male, 32 years old

omas of both types may secrete mucine: this observation is in favor of the origin of this lesion from Rathke's cysts and the authors call this lesion "cystic craniopharyngiomas with secretory component."

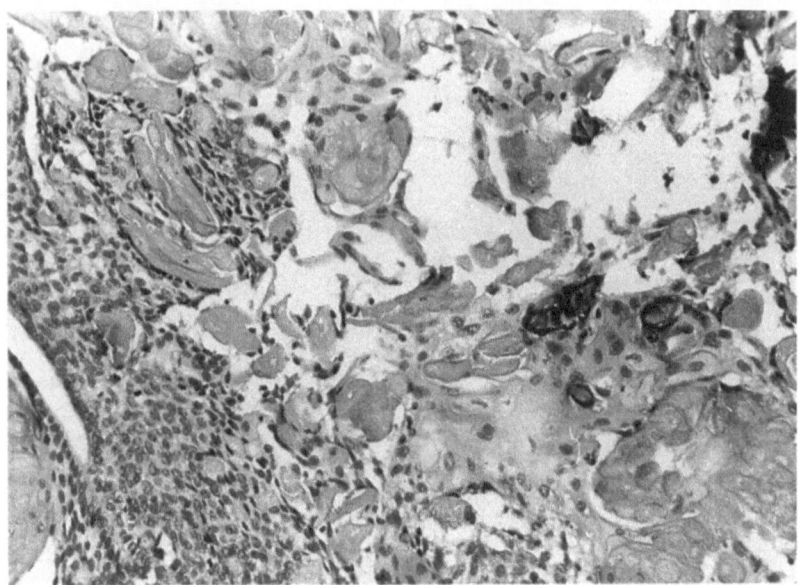

Fig. 4. Adamantinomatous craniopharyngioma. H & E, x140

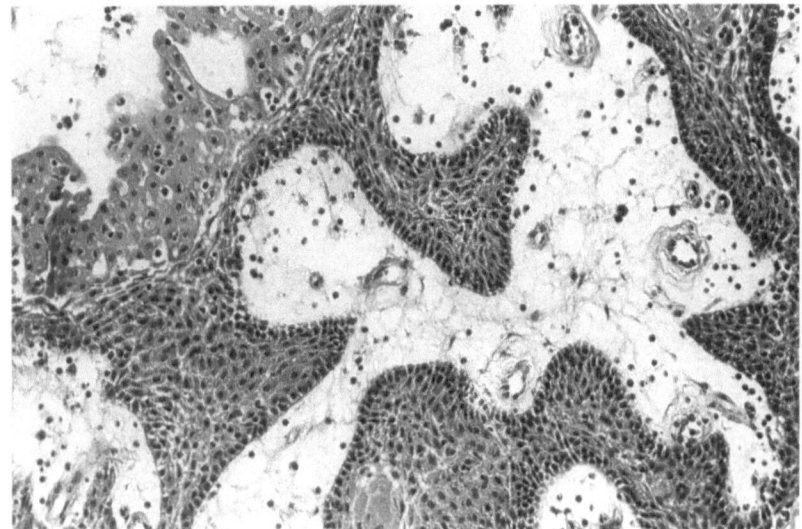

Fig. 5. Papillary craniopharyngioma. H & E, x180

Besides Liszczak et al. (1978), on the basis of morphological, biochemical, ultrastructural, and tissue culture studies performed on 25 cases of human craniopharyngiomas, supplied evidence to distinguish craniopharyngiomas in the typical, atypical and aggressive forms.

A common observation in both types is the reactive gliosis, sometimes marked, with Rosenthal's fibers of the nervous tissue when invaded by the lesion. Similar findings on small intraoperative biopsies can be erroneously interpreted as pilocytic astrocytoma.

Malignant transformation of craniopharyngiomas is exceptional. Nelson et al. (1988) describe, in a 49-year-old woman, a case of a suprasellar adamantinomatous craniopharyngioma operated on at the age of 35 which recurred and was submitted to radiotherapy when she was 42.

The prognosis of papillary craniopharyngioma is more favorable. Szeifert et al. (1993), in a study of 131 cases, observed 59% of recurrences in adamantinomatous craniopharyngiomas, 36% in those of the mixed type, and no recurrences in those of the papillary type.

References

Akimura T, Kameda H, Abiko S et al (1984) Infrasellar craniopharyngioma. Neuroradiology 31:180-183

Altinors S, Senvall E, Erdogan A et al (1984) Craniopharyngioma of the cerebellopontine angle. J Neurosurg 60:842-844

Burger PC, Vogel FS (1982) Surgical pathology of the nervous system and its covering, 2nd edn. Wiley, New York

Cooper PR, Ransohoff J (1972) Craniopharyngioma originating in the sphenoid bone: case report. J Neurosurg 36:102-106

Giangaspero F, Burger PC, Osborne DR, Stein RB (1984) Suprasellar papillary squamous epithelioma ("papillary craniopharyngioma"). Am J Surg Pathol 8:57-64

Hoffman HJ, De Silva M, Humphreys RP, Drake JM, Smith ML, Blaser SI (1992) Aggressive surgical management of craniopharyngiomas in children. J Neurosurg 76:47-52

Liszczak T, Richardson EP, Phillips JP, Jacobson S, Kornblith PL (1978) Morphological, biochemical, ultrastructural, tissue culture and clinical observations of typical and aggressive craniopharyngiomas. Acta Neuropathol (Berl) 43:191-203

Majlessi H, Shariat AS, Katirai A (1978) Nasopharyngeal craniopharyngioma: case report. J Neurosurg 49:119-120

Nelson GA, Bastian FO, Schlitt M, White RL (1988) Malignant transformation in craniopharyngioma. Neurosurgery 22:427-429

Petito Ck, De Girolami U, Earle KM (1976) Craniopharyngiomas: a clinical and pathological review. Cancer 37:1944-1952

Russel DS, Rubinstein LJ (1971) Pathology of tumours of the nervous system, 3rd edn. Williams and Wilkins, Baltimore

Russel DS, Rubinstein LJ (1977) Pathology of tumours of the nervous system. 4th edn. Williams and Wilkins, Baltimore

Szeifert GT, Pasztor E (1993) Could craniopharyngiomas produce pituitary hormones? Neurol Res 15:68-69

Szeifert GT, Julow J, Szabolski M, Slowik F, Balint K, Pasztor E (1991) Secretory component of cystic craniopharyngiomas: a mucino-histochemical and electronmicroscopic study. Surg Neurol 36:286-293

Szeifert GT, Sipos L, Horvath M, Sarker MH, Major O, Salomvary B, Czirjak S, Balint K, Slowik F, Kolonics L, Pasztor E (1993) Pathological characteristics of surgically removed craniopharyngiomas: analysis of 131 cases. Acta Neurochir (Wien) 124:139-143

Tachibana O, Yamashima T, Yamashita J, Takabatake Y (1994) Immunohistochemical expression of human chorionic gonadotropin and P glycoprotein in human pituitary glands and craniopharyngiomas. J Neurosurg 80:79-84

Neuroradiology of Craniopharyngiomas

M. Savoiardo and E. Ciceri

Craniopharyngiomas are solid and cystic tumors derived from remnants of the hypophyseal duct which usually grow in the suprasellar region; they also often grow in the sella turcica, and, much more rarely, in the third ventricle or in the sphenoid bone. They originate, therefore, along this midline axis, but they may extend, particularly with their cystic components, laterally into the middle fossa, anteriorly into the subfrontal region, and posteriorly into the posterior fossa.

In the general population, the incidence of craniopharyngioma is 3% of all intracranial tumors. More than 50% of these tumors develop in childhood and adolescence; they demonstrate a bimodal age distribution with one peak between age 5 and 10 and a second peak in the fifth-sixth decade. This is important because in the differential diagnosis of a suspected craniopharyngioma we have to consider different tumors according to age at presentation.

In the neuroradiological discussion of craniopharyngiomas, we must consider several different issues: (1) the role of different diagnostic techniques in the location and characterization of the tumor, (2) differential diagnosis, and (3) neuroradiological follow-up. A careful, critical analysis of postoperative results may improve surgical planning in future cases.

Neuroradiological Diagnosis

The neuroradiological evaluation of a craniopharyngioma is made with computed tomography (CT) or, even better, with magnetic resonance imaging (MRI). Occasionally, skull X-ray films may be helpful.

Department of Neuroradiology, Istituto Nazionale Neurologico "C. Besta", Via Celoria 11, 20133 Milan, Italy

Skull X-Ray Films

The role of skull films in diagnosing craniopharyngiomas is now negligible. However, the presence of some sellar enlargement and erosion with calcifications in the sellar and suprasellar region may occasionally be seen in skull films taken for other reasons, for instance, for trauma, and may be diagnostic. In our practice, X-ray films are used, with digital subtraction, when a cyst of craniopharyngioma has to be punctured stereotactically and when the patency of a catheter in a cyst needs to be reestablished. For expanding cysts, sometimes water-soluble contrast medium is injected and the content of the cyst aspirated. The changes in size of the cyst can be easily monitored, and the absence of leakage of contrast medium may be verified if bleomycin has to be injected. This information can also be obtained by CT (Fig. 1).

Computed Tomography

CT is usually adequate for diagnosing a craniopharyngioma, although the full extension of the tumor and its relation to the surrounding anatomical structures are better demonstrated by MRI. The main advantage of CT, besides its greater availability, is its ability to demonstrate calcifications.

Calcifications are present in most craniopharyngiomas and may appear as tiny, gritty, hyperdense foci or large irregular masses in the solid part of the tumor or as thin, short lamellae in the wall of a cyst.

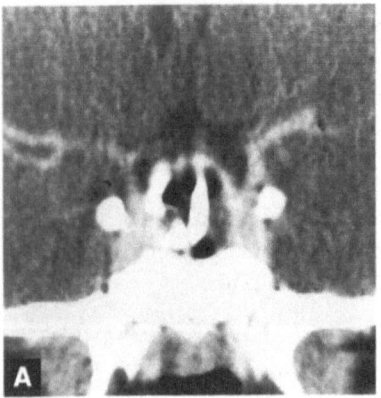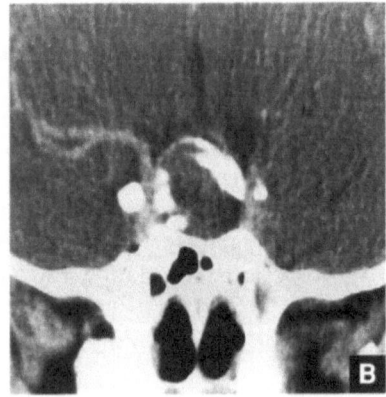

Fig. 1 A, B. CT scan, coronal sections, in a boy with a huge cystic craniopharyngioma treated with cyst aspiration and bleomycin at age 3. At age 5, the cyst is reaspirated and contains bubbles of air (**A**). Reexpansion of the cyst and increase of calcifications are demonstrated at age 7 (**B**)

The cystic components of the craniopharyngioma are often multiple and of variable size and density. They are usually hypodense with attenuation values slightly superior to those of the cerebrospinal fluid (CSF).

After contrast medium administration the solid component and the wall of the cysts enhance, thus allowing a better delineation of the tumor.

Magnetic Resonance Imaging

MRI obviously delineates the craniopharyngioma better on coronal and sagittal sections. With its various sequences, it separates the solid and cystic compartments neatly. Sometimes, however, the most reliable criteria for defining a cyst remain the homogeneity of the signal intensity and its smooth, rounded margins.

One characteristic feature of a considerable number of craniopharyngiomas is the high intensity signal of the cysts in Tl-weighted images (Fig. 2). However, cysts with different signal intensity may coexist, and the same cyst may change signal intensity in a short time (Fig. 3). Since cholesterol is known to be present in the cysts of craniopharyngiomas, it was thought to be responsible for this Tl-weighted, hyperintense signal (Pusey et al. 1987). However, a very accurate quantitative analysis of the cystic fluid of these tumors conducted by Ahmadi et al. (1992) demonstrated that cholesterol and triglyceride did not increase signal intensity. The high signal intensity in Tl-weighted images was caused by the presence of methemoglobin, a protein concentration greater than or equal to 9000 mg/dl, or both.

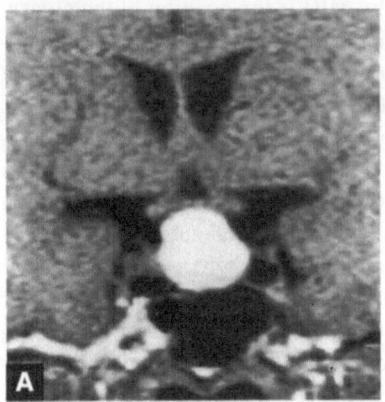 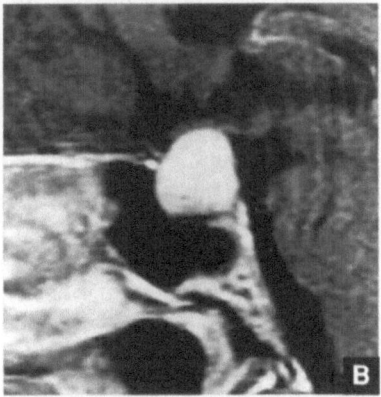

Fig. 2 A, B. Coronal (**A**) and sagittal (**B**) MR Tl-weighted sections of an intra- and suprasellar craniopharyngioma which slightly impinges upon the chiasm. The cystic component is markedly hyperintense. Mild hypointensity of the solid part is barely recognizable within the sella in the inferior part of the tumor

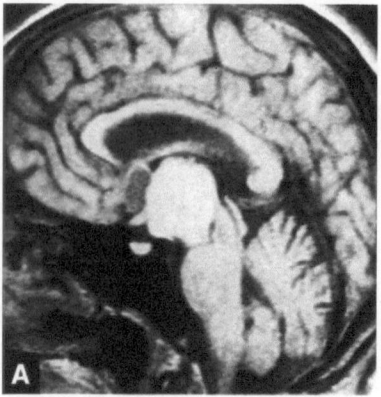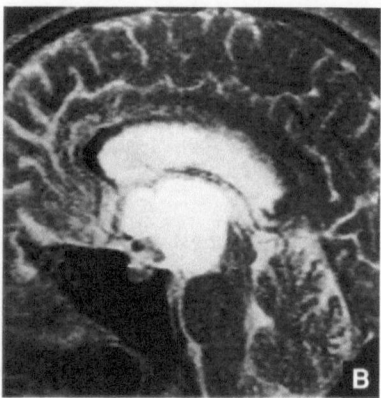

Fig. 3 A, B. Multicystic craniopharyngioma. **A** The Tl-weighted image shows a hypo-intense anterior cyst and a hyperintense larger posterior one. **B** In the T2-weighted image, both cysts are hyperintense

In craniopharyngiomas with high signal intensity in Tl- or in T2-weighted images, the size of the cyst may be overestimated with a standard window setting. Sometimes, only by adjusting the window can one recognize tiny septa or small peripheral solid components of the tumor (Fig. 4). Recognition of the solid component may be even easier after contrast medium administration (Fig. 5). Calcifications may escape detection by MRI, particularly when they are small, and CT in these cases may add specificity to the diagnosis.

One question that is usually solved by MRI is the position of the chiasm relative to the tumor. Sagittal and coronal sections are usually the most helpful, while axial sections, in the most common craniopharyngiomas of about 3 cm in diameter, demonstrate more clearly the lateral bowing of the optic tracts which are displaced and stretched by the tumor. When the optic chiasm is not clearly recognizable in the midline sagittal section, its position can usually be inferred from the position and inclination of the intracranial segment of the optic nerves seen on the adjacent lateral cuts (Fig. 6).

We have already mentioned the different locations where a craniopharyngioma may grow and the various extensions that it may present. In terms of differential diagnosis, it is obvious that craniopharyngiomas in rare locations, such as intrasphenoidal or intraventricular ones (Fig. 7), may be difficult to diagnose, and that a specific diagnosis may be reached sometimes only at surgery or at histological examination.

We shall now examine the most common differential diagnoses of a sellar and suprasellar tumor, separating them according to the typical age peaks of occurrence of craniopharyngiomas.

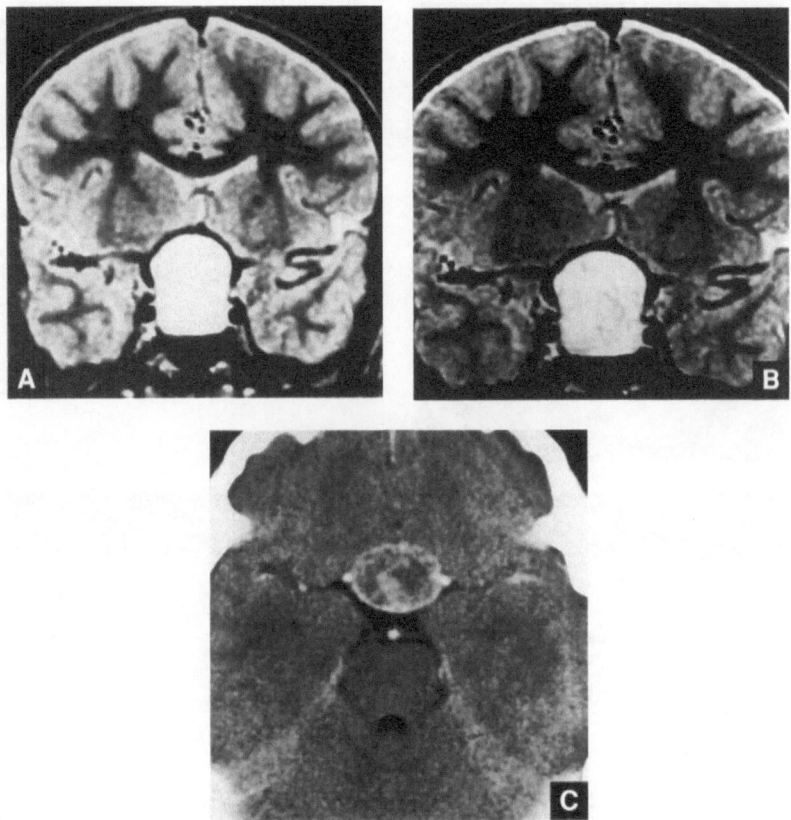

Fig. 4 A-C. Coronal T2-weighted image with standard window setting (**A**) shows homogeneous high signal intensity consistent with a large cyst. With a different window setting (**B**), several trabeculae are recognisable. They are also visible on the enhanced CT scan (**C**)

Differential Diagnosis

In childhood and adolescence, the tumors that must be considered more frequently in the differential diagnosis are chiasmatic and hypothalamic glioma and suprasellar ectopic germinoma; more rarely, Langerhans cell histiocytosis has to be considered.

Up to 45% of *chiasmatic gliomas* occur in patients with neurofibromatosis type 1 and often extend along the anterior optic pathways, either in the optic nerves or along the optic tracts, or both (Savoiardo et al. 1981); therefore, even disregarding density on CT or signal intensity on MRI and the absence of cysts and calcifications, they are usually easily identified. In contrast we have had problems in diagnosing correctly a few large *hypothalamic gliomas* which

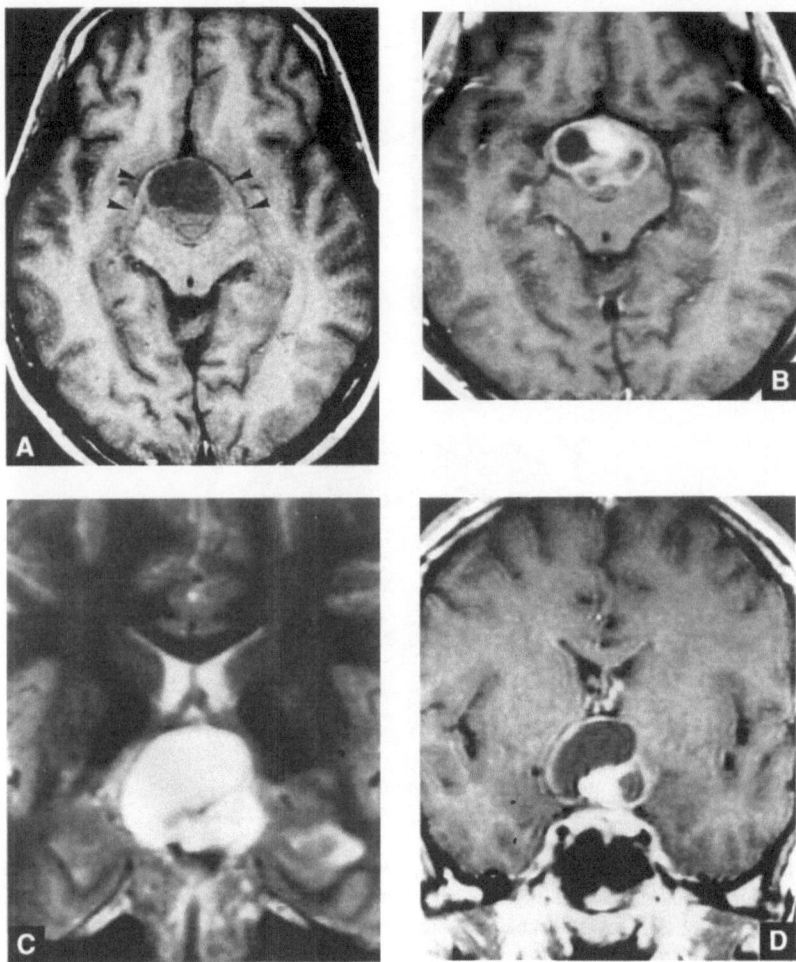

Fig. 5 A-D. Axial Tl-weighted image (**A**) fails to demonstrate the solid component of a craniopharyngioma which causes lateral bowing of the optic tracts (*arrowheads*). The solid component is well demonstrated on the post-contrast scan (**B**). Comparison of coronal T2-weighted (**C**) with post-contrast Tl-weighted image (**D**) also demonstrates better delineation of the solid component in the post-contrast MR image

involved the chiasm and the whole suprasellar region, with cystic extension into the posterior fossa and with a few calcifications that turned out to be pilocytic hypothalamic-chiasmatic gliomas at operation and histological examination. However, the growth pattern, the characteristics of signal intensity, and the absence of calcifications almost always allow easy differentiation of a hypothalamic glioma from craniopharyngioma (Fig. 8).

Hamartomas of the tuber cinereum usually do not create problems of differential diagnosis because of their typical site of origin, their pedunculated inferior extension, and their similarity to gray matter in density and signal intensity, although they may appear moderately hyperintense in proton density and T2-weighted images.

The *suprasellar germinoma* is easily diagnosed when the most common location in the pineal region is also present. When only the suprasellar mass is visible, it appears as a solid mass without cysts, enveloping the pituitary

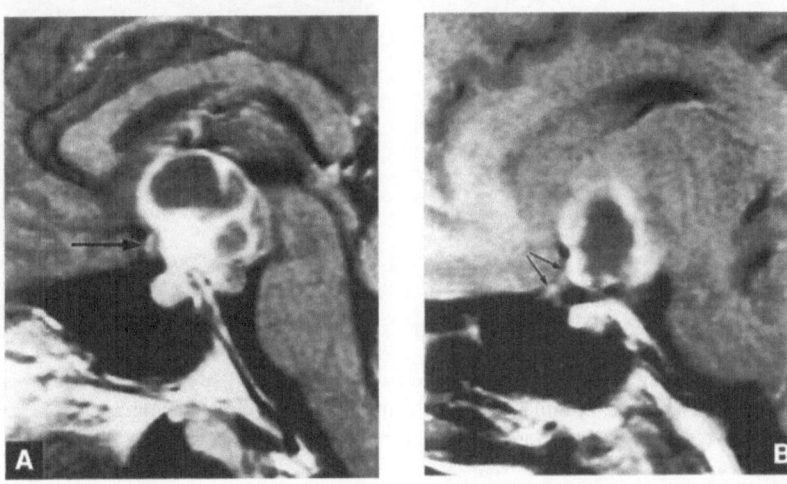

Fig. 6. A Midline sagittal section shows mild anterior and superior displacement of the chiasm (*arrow*). **B** A slightly more lateral section demonstrates the right elevated optic nerve (*arrows*), thus confirming the position of the chiasm

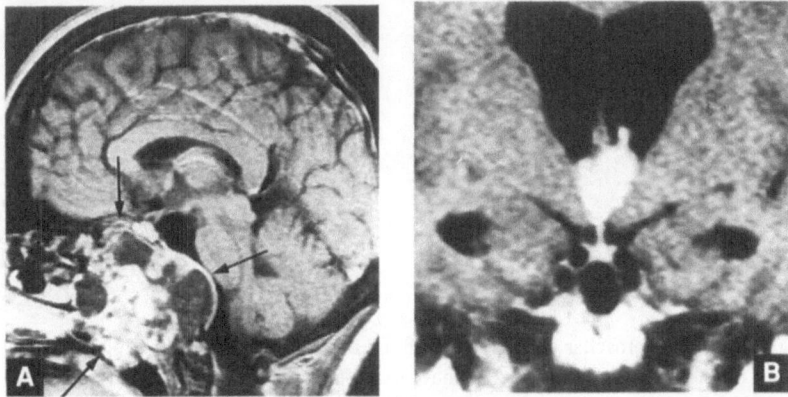

Fig. 7 A, B. Rare locations of craniopharyngiomas: intrasphenoidal (midline sagittal section, *arrows*, **A**), and intraventricular (coronal section, **B**). The sella and suprasellar cisterns are free of tumor in both cases

stalk, and impinging upon the antero-inferior profile of the third ventricle, often extending into the sella with a dumbbell shape narrowed at the level of the sellar diaphragm (Fig. 9). It is slightly hyperdense on CT and tends to be isointense to gray matter on MRI even in T2-weighted images, as is the case in all tumors with high cellularity, characterized by cells with a high nuclear-cytoplasmatic ratio. It may spread through the CSF, and a tiny enhancing

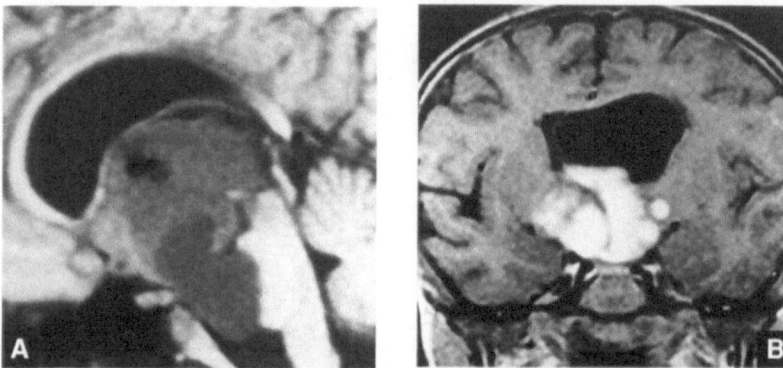

Fig. 8 A, B. Large hypothalamic pilocytic astrocytoma in sagittal (**A**) and coronal post-contrast (**B**) Tl-weighted images may be confused with a craniopharyngioma. Smudging of the enhancement toward the basal ganglia favors the diagnosis of glioma

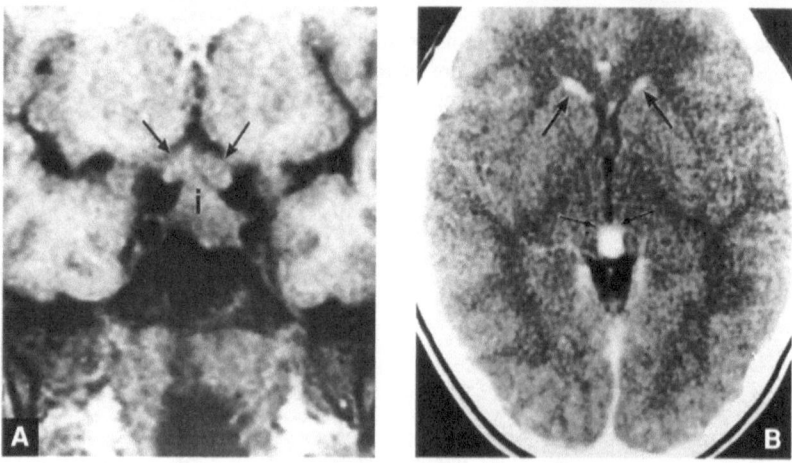

Fig. 9 A, B. Suprasellar germinoma with a dumbbell shape (**A**), encasing the pituitary infundibulum (*i*) and the chiasm (*arrows*), in a coronal Tl-weighted image. No pineal location was present in this case. In a different patient, a suprasellar mass could be diagnosed as a germinoma because of the slight enhancement on CT around the calcified pineal body (*thin arrows*) and the ependymal spread in the frontal horns (*thick arrows*, **B**)

rim along the profile of the frontal horns was the most common finding in such cases (Fig. 9). When the suprasellar germinoma is small, it may appear as a cone-shaped thin mass enveloping the infundibulum, down from the median eminence (Tien et al. 1991).

A similarly thin enhancement of a thickened infundibulum may be seen in *Langerhans cell histiocytosis* (Tien et al. 1990). Other locations of the disease, mainly in the bones, may lead to the correct diagnosis.

In adults, the differential diagnosis may include some pituitary adenomas and Rathke's cleft cysts. *Pituitary adenomas* can be confused with craniopharyngiomas only in a few situations, when they present with a prevailing suprasellar growth, particularly if they are hemorrhagic with a hyperintense signal in Tl-weighted images.

Rathke's cleft cysts have the same origin as craniopharyngiomas, from the remnants of an ectodermal structure, Rathke's pouch. They are a frequent incidental finding at autopsy, being observed in up to 30% of the post-mortem examinations (Okazaki and Scheithauer 1988). In this case, they are tiny cysts which bulge up from the intermediate lobe of the pituitary gland, just anterior to the infundibulum. When they enlarge, as they rarely do, they may cause symptoms and signs by compressing the surrounding structures. Their wall is a single-cell-layer epithelium and their content is similar to CSF in about half of the cases (Kucharczyk et al. 1987). However, the fluid of Rathke's cleft cysts may become creamy and waxy nodules may form on the wall; in these cases the density and the signal intensity change and differentiation from craniopharyngioma may become impossible. This is particularly true when the cyst is hyperintense in Tl-weighted images (Fig. 10). In addition, it has to be noted that transitional forms from Rathke's cleft cyst to craniopharyngioma do exist, with cysts partly lined by a single-cell-layer and partly by a stratified, squamous epithelium (Russell and Rubinstein 1989). We have also observed a patient in whom Rathke's cleft cyst was initially diagnosed at surgery who, at recurrence of the lesion, was found to have a craniopharyngioma with a cyst wall still consistent with a Rathke's cleft cyst (Fig. 10).

Other rare suprasellar lesions may occasionally enter into the differential diagnosis, as we have seen, for instance, in a case of *meningioma of the dorsum sellae* (Fig. 11); in this case, the vascularity of the tumor recognizable on MRI allowed the correct diagnosis.

Neuroradiological Follow-up and Conclusions

MRI with and without contrast administration is the best method for following up craniopharyngiomas to check for residual tumor after surgery or tumor recurrence even after an apparently complete removal. Sometimes CT

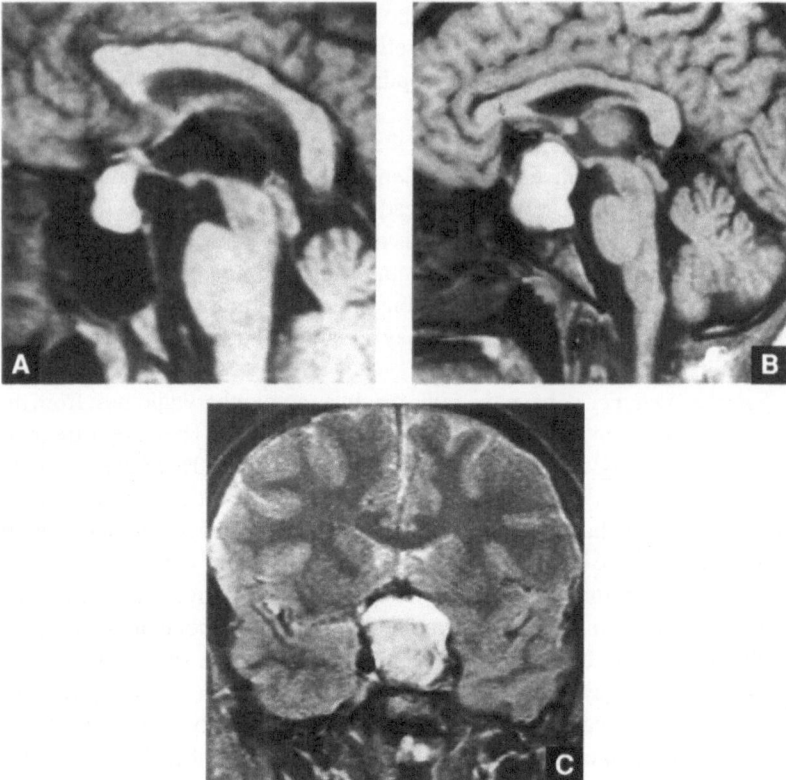

Fig. 10 A-C. Rathke's cleft cyst. There is high signal intensity in the T1-weighted image (**A**). In a different patient, already operated for Rathke's cleft cyst, a recurrence has similar signal intensity in T1-weighted image (**B**), but inhomogeneous signal intensity in the coronal T2-weighted image (**C**). At operation, craniopharyngioma tissue in the inferior part of the tumor and a superior cyst with a single-cell-layered wall were found

is superior to MRI, by demonstrating a tiny residual calcification when MRI showed a complete removal.

Chances for completely removing a craniopharyngioma are greater in the first operation, particularly in small, solid, suprasellar tumors. Large multicystic tumors are difficult to remove, and recurrences are frequent even in the hands of the best neurosurgeons.

When residual tumor is demonstrated, it is often difficult to decide whether reoperation or stereotactic X-ray treatment is the best course of action. It may even be difficult to be sure whether minor postsurgical abnormalities represent scar tissue or residual tumor (Fig. 12). Sometimes the neurosurgeon knows that he has left some tumor tissue, for instance attached to the carotid siphon, and the neuroradiologist cannot recognize it.

In order to recognize possible residual tumor, the neuroradiologist must know how the operation was performed; the residual tumor is usually found in areas that are hidden in the approach that was used. For instance, in the anterolateral subfrontal, pterional approach, residual tumor is usually seen in the homolateral anterior part of the sella (Fig. 13). Removal of the anterior clinoid, as suggested by Dolenc, may allow greater access to the sella and complete removal of the tumor. In the anterior midline approach, with sectioning of the anterior communicating artery, large tumors may be removed, but a tiny portion behind the tuberculum sellae may be left (Fig. 13). Sometimes a transcallosal or a bilateral approach, as indicated by Choux et al. (this volume), is necessary for removing large tumors.

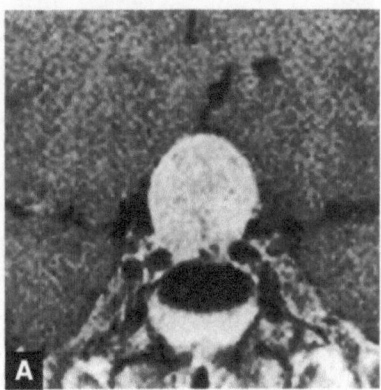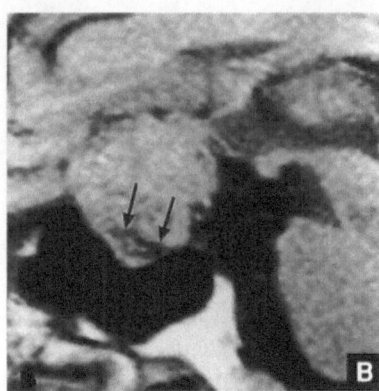

Fig. 11 A, B. Postcontrast coronal (**A**) and sagittal without contrast (**B**) T1-weighted images of a sellar and suprasellar mass. Visualization of tumor vessels in the unenhanced MR scan (*arrows*, **B**) allows the diagnosis of meningioma of the dorsum sellae

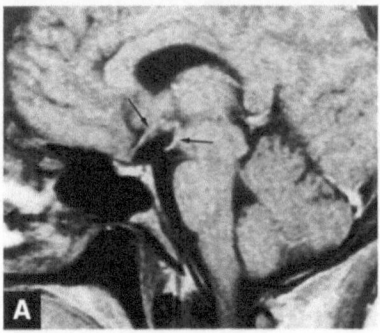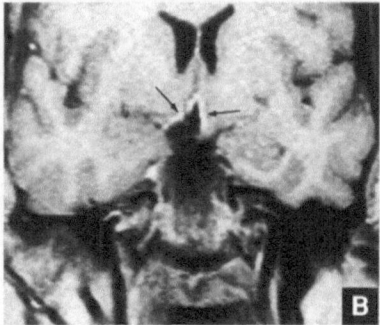

Fig. 12 A, B. Sagittal (**A**) and coronal (**B**) postcontrast MR images, after apparently complete removal of a 4-cm craniopharyngioma, show a thin rim of enhancement (*arrows*) in the chiasmatic-hypothalamic region: glial scar or residual tumor? The findings are unchanged at 2-year follow-up

Neuroradiologists and neurosurgeons sometime disagree about the presence of cysts in craniopharyngiomas. The neurosurgeon may complain that a tumor indicated as cystic was almost entirely solid at operation. This simply depends on the different emphasis that they put on the presence of cysts; the neuroradiologist uses the cysts as a reliable element for the differential diagnosis and describes them even if they are small, of no importance for the

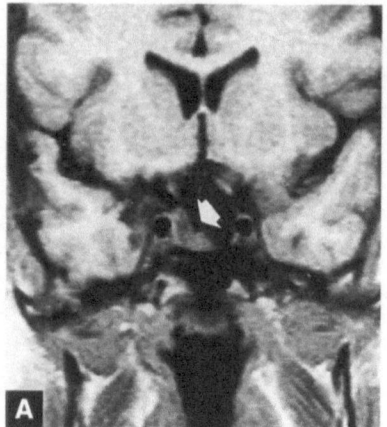 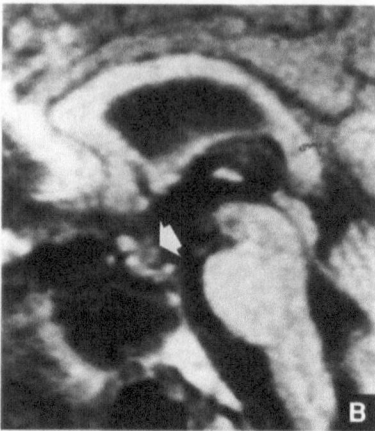

Fig. 13 A, B. Postoperative MR studies in two different patients with large craniopharyngiomas. Coronal Tl-weighted image in a patient operated via a right subfrontal pterional approach (**A**) shows residual tumor in the right anterior part of the sella (*arrow*). The sagittal section in a patient operated via an anterior approach (**B**) demonstrates a tiny residual tumor (*arrow*) hidden by the tuberculum sellae

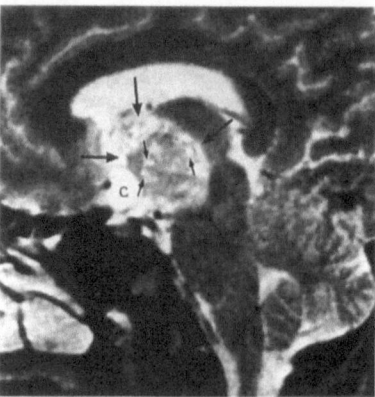

Fig. 14. Sagittal T2-weighted image of a large, solid craniopharyngioma (*long arrows*), with an anterior inferior cyst (*c*). The numerous small hyperintense areas also consistent with cysts (*short arrows*) are of diagnostic importance, but irrelevant for surgery

neurosurgeon during the operation, because opening them does not debulk the tumor (Fig. 14). Careful analysis of the images and a close collaboration between the neuroradiologist and the neurosurgeon are necessary in planning surgery, in recognizing pitfalls, and in locating the residual tumor in order to improve the surgical approach in the future.

References

Ahmadi J, Destian S, Apuzzo MLJ, Segall HD, Zee CS (1992) Cystic fluid in craniopharyngiomas: MR imaging and quantitative analysis. Radiology 182:783-785

Kucharczyk W, Peck WW, Kelly WM, Norman D, Newton TH (1987) Rathke cleft cysts: CT, MR imaging, and pathologic features. Radiology 165:491-495

Okazaki H, Scheithauer BW (1988) Atlas of neuropathology. Gower, New York

Pusey E, Kortman KE, Flannigan BD, Tsuruda J, Bradley WG (1987) MR of craniopharyngiomas: tumor delineation and characterization. AJNR 8:439-444

Russell DS, Rubinstein LJ (1989) Pathology of tumours of the nervous system, 5th edn. Arnold, London

Savoiardo M, Harwood-Nash DC, Tadmor R, Scotti G, Musgrave MA (1981) Gliomas of the intracranial anterior optic pathways in children. Radiology 138:601-610

Tien RD, Newton TH, McDermott MW, Dillon WP, Kucharczyk J (1990) Thickened pituitary stalk on MR images in patients with diabetes insipidus and Langerhans cell histiocytosis. AJNR 11:703-708

Tien R, Kucharczyk J, Kucharczyk W (1991) MR imaging of the brain in patients with diabetes insipidus. AJNR 12:533-542

Craniopharyngioma in Children: Surgical Considerations

M. Choux, G. Lena, and L. Genitori

The management of craniopharyngiomas, especially in childhood, remains a controversial and challenging subject (Carmel et al. 1982; Fischer et al. 1985; Katz 1975; Yasargil et al. 1990). This histologically benign tumor is of maldevelopmental origin and develops in a particular intracranial location, close to the optic pathways, the hypothalamus, the hypophysis, and the internal carotid arteries and their main branches. Its spontaneous evolution is unforeseeable. The location and firm attachment to important surrounding anatomical structures make its surgical extirpation possible, but difficult and risky. Other therapeutic modalities have been proposed, such as conventional or interstitial irradiation or even chemotherapy. The choice of one or another treatment depends on the patient's age, the aspects of the lesion, the skyll of the surgeon, and, moreover, the personal opinion and the firm belief of the physician. Consequently, it is not so easy to establish a definitive protocol for the management of craniopharyngioma. We have tried in this presentation to present our personal therapeutic approach to this tumor, considering exclusively the pediatric age.

A personal series of 54 craniopharyngiomas treated since 1975 in patients under the age of 16 in our department is presented and compared with a cooperative series of 474 pediatric craniopharyngiomas collected from members of the French-speaking Neurosurgical Society and colleagues from the International Society for Pediatric Neurosurgery. These data were published in a monograph in 1991 (Choux et al. 1991). We will point out in this presentation exclusively what our personal surgical considerations are. We do not discuss clinical or radiological data.

Patients

Age and initial clinical manifestations must be taken into consideration when surgical management is discussed. In this series of 474 pediatric cases, age

Department of Pediatric Neurosurgery, Hôpital des Enfants, La Timone Marseille, France distribution is as follows: 3.8% were under the age of 2; 19.2% between 3 and 5 years; the majority, 40%, between 6 and 10; and 24.5% between 11 and 16 years. We note that a quarter of craniopharyngiomas are discovered in children under the age of 5. Management is significantly different in young and in older patients.

The diagnosis delay varies in most of the cases from 13 to 20 months, but we have patients who presented with an initial growth failure many years before the diagnosis. The main presenting symptoms are raised intracranial pressure in 60%-75% of the cases, visual disturbances in 50%, and endocrine dysfunctions in 15%-20% of the cases, mainly growth failure or diabetes insipidus. Panhypopituitarism at presentation is not rare and only 9%-29% of children have normal endocrine function. Hydrocephalus is present in 30% of cases.

The Tumor

We have confirmed in this series of 474 cases that in children a craniopharyngioma is nearly always of the adamantinomatous type.

Three main *tumoral aspects* are observed. Solid tumors represent only 9%. Mainly cystic tumors are less frequent in children (36%) than in adults. At the pediatric age, the majority (55%) are mixed tumors. From a surgical point of view we have observed that mixed tumors are easier to dissect and remove than purely solid tumors. Exclusively cystic lesions, especially in young patients, may be possibly considered for other treatments, such as interstitial irradiation or intracystic bleomycin injection.

Considering the *volume*, we have seen in this series as well as in the literature that craniopharyngiomas in children are more commonly larger than in adults (more than 3 cm in 80% of the cases). Giant tumors in our series and in the literature, too, are mainly described in children and especially in young children (Ammirati et al. 1990).

Topographically, the craniophayngioma may have a single or combined localization. In 50% a single localization was found: retrochiasmatic (21%), prechiasmatic (17.5%), intrasellar (8%), and intraventricular (3.5%). This anatomical classification may be criticized, since exclusively prechiasmatic lesions are exceptional. Most of them are retrochiasmatic with a more or less important prechiasmatic extension. True intraventricular craniopharyngiomas exist, even if they are exceptional. A large proportion of craniopharyngiomas in children are both intrasellar and prechiasmatic (13%), retrochiasmatic (5.5%), or pre-and retrosellar (5.5%). Consequently, we may say that in children 32% of craniopharyngiomas involve the intrasellar region. We must note that in this series 4.2% of the lesion extended posteriorly in the posterior fossa.

Treatment

Five therapeutic modalities for craniopharyngiomas may be proposed and discussed: surgery, conventional irradiation, interstitial irradiation, radiosurgery, and chemotherapy. Personally, we recommend surgery as initial treatment in almost all of the pediatric cases we deal only with. In very few cases (a young child with a small craniopharyngioma, presenting no or only mild endocrinological symptoms and no visual signs), an aggressive treatment may be delayed, watching and looking for a clinical development in conjunction with regular magnetic resonance imaging (MRI) control. We have followed three young patients for more 2 years without significant clinical modifications, growing normally, and without endocrinological worsening. Except these, very particular cases, most of the pediatric patients we see are operated on with the goal to totally remove the lesion in one step without mortality and without an intolerable morbidity.

In the *preoperative period* complete endocrinological investigation and preparation are needed. The surgical protocol is established with computed tomographic (CT) scan and MRI only. For 10 years now we have not asked for routine preoperative angiography. MRI alone allows one to choose the best surgical approach and prepares the neurosurgeon for the complex procedure (Fig. 1).

Hydrocephalus is frequently associated (in 44.54% of 341 patients in the literature and in 42.5% in our cooperative series). Hydrocephalus is more frequently found in children than in adults. An initial shunt was implanted in 33.7% of 294 patients reported in the literature and in 29% of our series. In a significant number of patients a secondary shunt is needed. In a series of 357

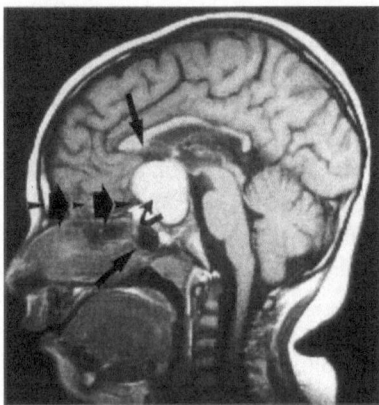

Fig. 1. Surgical protocol from MRI only. Different and combined surgical approaches and possible relationships with optic pathways and hypothalamus can be established using MRI alone

cases a definitive shunt existed in 27.7% of the children. We try to remove the tumor without routine shunt implantation and restrict shunting to very young patients presenting with acute, and severe hydrocephalus.

Surgical Anatomy

In few publications a *presurgical biopsy* has been proposed. We do not see any indication for a biopsy in cases of suspected craniopharyngioma.

Before describing the different surgical approaches we must consider the *seven critical surgical points* we need to know beforehand: the relationships of the tumor with the hypothalamus and the third ventricle, the optic pathways, the hypophysis, the pituitary stalk the vessels, the brainstem, and the dura.

1) Craniopharyngioma and the Hypothalamus

Preoperatively, it is generally difficult to predict what degree of adherence there will be between the capsule of the tumor and the floor of the third ventricle. It is one of the key points when we consider the limitation of a total removal or when we want to avoid major postoperative morbidity. Few interesting reports have illustrated these relationships: Ciric in 1977 and Steno in 1985. The existence of gliosis between the tumor and the brain is controversial. Though not admitted by some authors, this glial layer is accepted by others. Sweet (1988) has written: "The functionless glia may provide a significant margin of safety between the growing epithelial cells to be excised and the vitally important thalamo-hypothalamic and visual structures that should be preserved intact". We are convinced that in many cases a craniopharyngioma may be separated from the floor of the third ventricle without injuring the hypothalamus. The capsule of the tumor invaginates the neural tissue but may be gently separated by pushing down the tumoral capsule. During surgery it is better to preserve intact a large portion of the capsule such that it can be pulled on it in one piece (Fig. 2).

2) Craniopharyngiomas and the Optic Pathways

Frequently compressed, optic pathways must be initially located and separated from the capsule. Even in cases of apparently nonvisible optic nerves or chiasma, when the cyst is empty, it is nearly always possible to dissect them. Exceptionally intrachiasmatic craniopharyngiomas have been described. The main risk here is secondary deterioration of visual acuity when the optic pathways have been compressed for a long period of time or in cases of microtrauma during surgical dissection. In severe preoperative visual disturbances we recommend decompressing the tumor in a first step, puncturing a cyst, for example, and waiting a few days before removing the tumor.

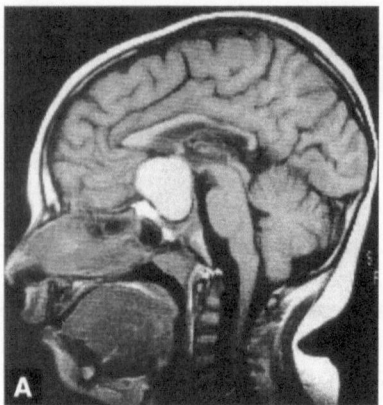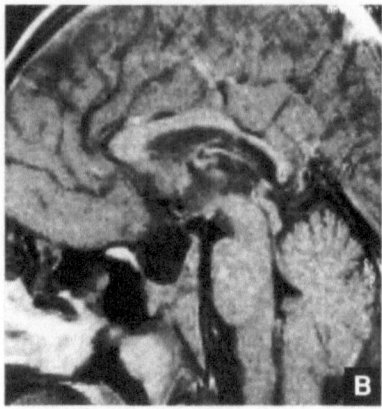

Fig. 2 A, B. Preoperative (**A**) and postoperative (**B**) MRI, showing a total removal of a craniopharyngioma with preservation of the hypothalamus

3) Craniopharyngiomas and the Pituitary Stalk

The pituitary stalk is not always visible during the procedure. Its preservation is a subject of controversy. It is clear in the series as well as in the literature that sectioning of the pituitary stalk is followed by secondary diabetes insipidus in 70% of the cases and its preservation by only 35%. It is easier to preserve it using the pterional route (56%) than the subfrontal approach (36%). We agree with Hoffman et al. (1977): "The very nature of the tumor necessitates sacrifice of the pituitary stalk". Its preservation will increase the rate of recurrence, since the tumor more or less involves the stalk and removal of the tumor will be more limited. Consequently, we have the choice between proceeding with total removal, which involves sections of the stalk, or preserving the stalk, which means tumor resection is incomplete. Personally, our choice is clear and we always adopt the first option.

4) Craniopharyngiomas and the Vessels

Adherences between the tumoral capsule and the vessels, mainly the carotid artery or the anterior cerebral artery, are one of the main obstacles for a correct extirpation of the tumor. More difficult to manage are the vessels coming from the optic pathways and the hypothalamus which may be injured during the procedure. Vascular problems may be seen after surgery, such as postoperative aneurysms or dilatation. Though mentioned in the literature, we have never encountered such complications in our experience.

5) Craniopharyngioma and Brainstem

Close adherences between a craniopharyngioma and the brainstem are very rare. An arachnoidal sheath is nearly always present and we have never seen the tumoral capsule adhering to the basilar trunk. A giant craniopharyngioma may extend posteriorly, pushing back the brainstem or extending into the posterior fossa without invasion of the brainstem. Consequently, it is essential to know that a craniopharyngioma extensively developed posteriorly with deformation of the brainstem may be surgically removed without injuring the anatomical structures of the brainstem (Fig. 3).

6) Craniopharyngioma and Hypophysis

Except for intrasellar craniopharyngiomas, the hypophysis is not a real problem. It is generally pushed down into the sella by the tumor. We have never seen an ectopic hypophysis as it has been described in rare cases in the literature.

7) Craniopharyngioma and the Dura

Adherences with the dura are rare and always located at the level of the sella. In some cases, especially in a few intrasellar craniopharyngiomas, it may be difficult to separate the tumor capsule and the dura without opening the cavernous sinus. In these cases laser may be useful to burn the dural adherences. In infants large craniopharyngiomas may, though rarely, develop from the sellar region and extend superiorly, covered by the dura of the sella. Approaching the tumor subfrontally, the thick layer covering the lesion is the dura and not the tumoral capsule.

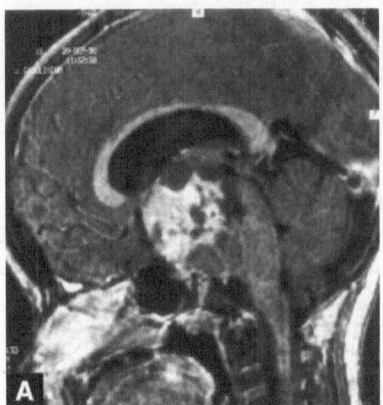 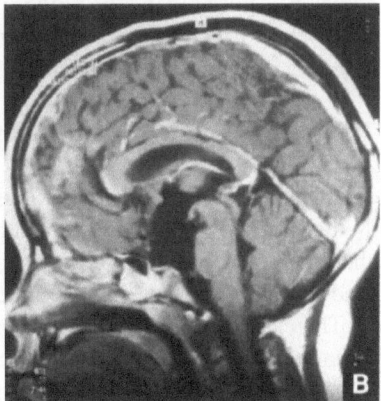

Fig. 3. A Preoperative MRI: large craniopharyngioma occupying the suprasellar region, invading the third ventricle and pushing the brainstem backward. **B** Postoperative MRI: total excision using a subfrontal approach and opening of the lamina terminalis. Brainstem returned to a normal aspect

Surgical Approach

Out of 415 cases, a single *surgical approach* was used in 89% of the cases: unilateral subfrontal (46%), pterional (27%), transsphenoidal (8%), trans-ventricular (3%), bilateral frontal (2.6%) and transcallosal (0.7%). We strongly recommend starting with unilateral or bilateral anterior approach. The rationale for this is that this approach provides a better bilateral view of the tumor, a complete estimation of its extension and the degree of compression of the optic pathways, and makes total extirpation of the lesion possible by coupling it with a bifrontal, pterional, or transcallosal approach. More and more now, we use a bilateral frontal approach, which allows a better control of both sides with possible preservation of both olfactory nerves. Conse-quently, the skin incision, which will be bicoronal, will allow adaptation and possibly extension of the initial bone flap to another approach during the same procedure. We do not recommend the transcallosal route as the only approach to remove a craniopharyngioma (Konovalov 1987). We restrict its use to cases of giant craniopharyngioma developed upward and used in com-bination with the anterior approach.

During the surgical procedure opening of the lamina terminalis may be useful. For us it is an essential technique in the management of craniopharyn-gioma. Removal of a retrochiasmatic lesion may be accomplished exclusively through the lamina terminalis. In most of the cases we open the lamina termi-nalis routinely at the end of procedure to make sure that the third ventricle is free and that we have totally resected the tumor (Lapras et al. 1987).

In the cooperative series of 454 cases total extirpation was possible in 55.3% and a subtotal extirpation in 38.7%. In our personal series, total re-moval was possible in 72% (Figs. 2 a, b, 3 a, b). In the prachiasmatic type a complete extirpation was possible in 73% and in the intrasellar type in 68%.

Radiation Treatment and Chemotherapy

At the pediatric age *irradiation* must be avoided, even in subtotal removal. In the last 10 years not one patient has been irradiated in our department. If there is residual tumor we prefer to wait and to observe the development. Radiosurgery may possibly be indicated in few cases.

There are some indications for *intracavitary irradiation* when the crani-opharyngioma is mainly cystic (Backlund et al. 1989). We do not have great experience with this technique in children.

In five cases during the last 3 years we have employed *intracavitary chem-otherapy* (Broggi et al. 1989), with injection of bleomycin. Indications are cystic tumor in patients with mild clinical symptoms. After 3 years of fol-low-up of our first case, a 5-year-old boy, the tumor has apparently disappeared and there have been no further clinical symptoms. Intracavitary treatment with bleomycin may be used as single treatment or as preliminary treatment before surgical removal of the tumor. In the latter shrinkage of the capsule will facilitate its dissection and removal.

Results

Survival

The general survival rate in this series is 89.5%.

Surgical Mortality

Surgical mortality (2 months) is 3.7%, with one death at 20 days of a patient with postoperative cerebral ischemia related to severe vasospasm of the middle cerebral artery and another death at 25 days due to metabolic disturbances. In craniopharyngiomas we consider that at least 2 months must be considered as the operative period.

Recurrence

In our experience the *recurrence* rate is 19.1% for patients who had a supposed total extirpation and 56.6% for those with subtotal extirpation. In children, surgery is the main step for management of first recurrence. The second operation is not usually much more complicated than the first one and we have seen in a few cases that total removal, which was considered impossible at the first operation, was accomplished during the second operation.

Functional Results

1) Visual Results
Age is not a prognostic factor concerning the visual outcome. But in very young children the delay between the first visual manifestation may be more important than in older patients. Moreover, an infant may present unilateral blindness which cannot be detected for a long period of time. The duration of preoperative symptoms is an important prognostic factor. In cases of severe preoperative visual deficit we recommend decompressing the optic pathways in a first stage before dissecting the tumor and removing it. It is clear that total removal of the lesion gives the best ophthalmological results.

2) Neurological Results

Postoperative neurological deficits are rare. Rates of epilepsy mentioned in the literature are between 1.7% (Shapiro et al. 1979) and 21.4% (Pierre-Kahn et al. 1988). In our cooperative series late epilepsy is described in 16% of the cases. The epilepsy was severe in 2%. More important is to study the psychological sequelae of the children operated on the degree of autonomy and the future quality of life (Cavazuti et al. 1983; Choux and Lena 1979; Pierre-Kahn 1988).

Autonomy. In 380 cases autonomy was assessed with the following results: total autonomy: 66%; moderate handicap: 17%; severe handicap: 8%; total dependence: 4%; and too young: 5%.

Education. We have studied the level of education in 383 cases: normal education: 63%; institution: 10%; special school: 9%; no school: 8%; university: 3%; too young: 7%.

Neuropsychological Outcome. Neuropsychological outcome was studied in 110 patients.

Modifications of behavior were found in more than 50% of the cases but they were important in only 15%. Hyperphagia has been described, associated in few cases with obesity, fury and dementia. Memory disorders were detected in 37% of the patients. In the majority of the cases these memory disorders are transitory. It is difficult to assess this complication in patients who cannot always be tested before surgery.

3) Endocrinological Results

After surgery, a worsening of endocrine functions is observed in all the cases: obesity (33%); diabetes insipidus (70%); and growth deficiency, even if paradoxical spontaneous growth is observed in 33% of the cases.

Biologically, deficits concern: growth hormone (95%), thyroid hormone (90%), adrenocorticotropic hormone (75%) and luteinizing hormone/follicle-stimulating hormone (95%). Only 5% of the children are endocrinologically intact.

It must be pointed out that late morbidity and even late mortality may be clearly related with endocrinological and metabolic problems.

Conclusion

In this study we have stressed the necessity to surgically remove a craniopharyngioma at the pediatric age as totally as possible during the first procedure. In our practice this goal is possible in 70% of the cases, with a very low operative mortality. In recent years morbidity has decreased significantly, even if the endocrinological results remain poor. The main risk in a child treated for a craniopharyngioma is recurrence and from the start the best must be done to prevent such recurrence.

References

Ammirati M, Samii M, Sephernis A (1990) Surgery of large retrochiasmatic craniopharyngioma in children. Childs Nerv Syst 6:13-17

Backlund EO, Axelsson B, Bergstrand CG, Eriksson AL, Noren G, Ribbesio E, Rahn T, Schnell PO, Tallstedt L, Saaf M, et al (1989) Treatment of craniopharyngiomas -the stereotactic approach in a ten to twenty-three years perspective. Surgical radiological and ophthalmological aspects. Acta Neurochir (Wien) 99:11-91

Broggi G, Giorgi C, Franzini A, Servello D, Solero CL (1989) Preliminary results of intracavitary treatment of craniopharyngiomas with bleomycin. J Neurosurg Sci 33:145-148

Carmel PW, Antunez JL, Chang CH (1982) Craniopharyngiomas in children. Neurosurgery 11:382-389

Cavazuti V, Fischer EG, Welch K (1983) Neurological and psychological sequelae following different treatments of craniopharyngioma in children. J Neurosurg 59:409

Choux M, Lena G (1979) Bases of surgical management of craniopharyngioma in children proceedings. Acta Neurochir Suppl (Wien) 28:348

Choux M, Lena G, Genitori L (1991) Le craniopharyngiome de l'Enfant. Neurochirurgie 37:1-174

Ciric I (1977) On the origin and nature of the pituitary gland capsule. J Neurosurg 46:596-600

Fischer EG, Welch K, Belli JA, Wallman J, Shillito J Jr, Winston KR, Cassady R (1985) Treatment of craniopharyngiomas in children (1972-1981). J Neurosurg 62:496-501

Hoffman HJ, Hendrick EB, Humphreys RP Buncic JR Armstrong DL, Jenkin RD (1977) Management of craniopharyngioma in children. J Neurosurg 47:218-227

Katz EL (1975) Late results of radical excision of craniopharyngiomas in children. J Neurosurg 47:86-93

Kobayashi T, Kageyama N, Ohara K (1981) Internal irradiation for cystic craniopharyngioma. J Neurosurg 55:896-903

Konovalov AN (1987) Technique and strategies of direct surgical management of craniopharyngiomas. In: Apuzzo M (ed) Surgery of the third ventricle. Williams and Wilkins, Baltimore, 542-552

Lapras C, Patet JD, Mottolese C, Gharbi S, Lapras C jr (1987) Craniopharyngiomas in childhood: analysis of 42 cases. Prog Exp Tumor Res 30:350-358

Laws ER jr (1980) Transsphenoidal microsurgery in the management of craniopharyngioma. J Neurosurg 52:661-666

Mori K, Handa H, Murata T, Takeuchi J, Miwa S, Osaka K (1980) Results of treatment for craniopharyngioma. Childs Brain 6:306-312

Pierre-Kahn A, Brauner R, Renier D, Sainte-Rose C, Gangemi MA, Rapport R, Hirsch JF (1988) Traitement des craniopharyngiomes de l'enfant. Analyse rétrospective de 50 observations. Arch Fr Pediatr 45:163-167

Raimondi AJ, Rougerie J (1983) A critical review of personal experiences with craniopharyngioma: clinical history, surgical techniques, and operative results. Conc Pediatr Neurosurg 3:1-34

Shapiro K, Till K, Grant DN (1979) Craniopharyngiomas in childhood. A rational approach to treatment. J Neurosurg 50:617-623

Shillito J jr (1986) Treatment of craniopharyngioma. Clin Neurosurg 33:533-546

Steno J (1985) Microsurgical topography of craniopharyngiomas. Acta Neurochir Suppl (Wien) 35:94-100

Sweet WH (1988) Craniopharyngiomas (with a note on Rathke's cleft or epithelial cyst and on suprasellar cyst). In: Schmidek HM, Sweet WH (ed) Operative neurosurgical techniques. Grune and Stratton, Orlando, pp 349-379

Symon L, Sprich W (1985) Radical excision of craniopharyngioma. Results in 20 patiens. J Neurosurg 62:174-181

Yasargil MG, Curcic M, Kis M, Siegenthaler G, Teddy PJ, Roth P (1990) Total removal of craniopharyngioma. Approach and long-term results in 144 patients. J Neurosurg 73:11

Radical Removal of Craniopharyngiomas 1971-1991

P. W. CARMEL

Introduction

Craniopharyngiomas are histologically benign tumors that may be lethal if incompletely treated. Our attempts at radical removal of these tumors owe much to the work of Dr. William Sweet (1988) who showed that the projections of tumor that extend into neural tissue are actually surrounded by a thick glial layer. Splitting of this glial layer permits removal of the tumor while preserving the neural structures.

This report details experience with 99 patients with craniopharyngiomas operated by the author at the Neurological Institute of New York between 1971 and 1991. This group included 72 children and 27 adults. Sixty-five of the patients had their first operation at the Neurological Institute, while 34 had been operated on initially elsewhere. This secondary operation group had undergone 46 prior operations and 18 had also received radiation therapy. These 99 patients underwent 133 operations at the Neurological Institute (excluding shunts, drains, etc). Fifteen patients had two operations, three patients had three operations, and two patients had more than three operations (Table 1).

Patients, Methods, and Results

While the goal of therapy in most of these patients was the complete removal of tumor, I believe that it is not possible to totally remove all craniopharyngiomas. This limitation is illustrated by the first case, an 11-year-old boy with a cystic, partially calcified tumor (Fig. 1). Figure 2 is an operative view of his right optic nerve. This nerve was still functioning despite decreased acuity and hemianopic field cut. Good visualization of the nerve under the operating microscope showed dense calcification with no observable separation from the nerve, and I did not feel that this calcification could be re-

University of Medicine and Dentistry of New Jersey, 90 Bergen Street, Newark, New Jersey 07103, USA

moved without seriously damaging his vision. A calcified remnant was seen on postoperative computed tomographic (CT) scans (Fig. 3). This residual calcification was monitored by scan for almost 4 years, when visible soft-tissue growth prompted the use of radiation therapy.

During 65 primary operations, total removal was achieved in 45 patients (69%), with slightly higher success in children than adults (Table 2). There is a marked and perhaps necessary learning curve in accomplishing this re-

Table 1. Craniopharyngioma 1971-1991

Patients	(n)
Total	99
• Children	72
• Adults	27
Patients, primary operation	65
Patients, secondary operation	34
Operations at NINY	
Total	133 [a]
Patients, two operations	15
Patients, three operations	3
More than three operations	2
Operations prior to treatment at NINY	46 [a]

NINY, Neurological Institute of New York
[a] Excludes shunts etc.

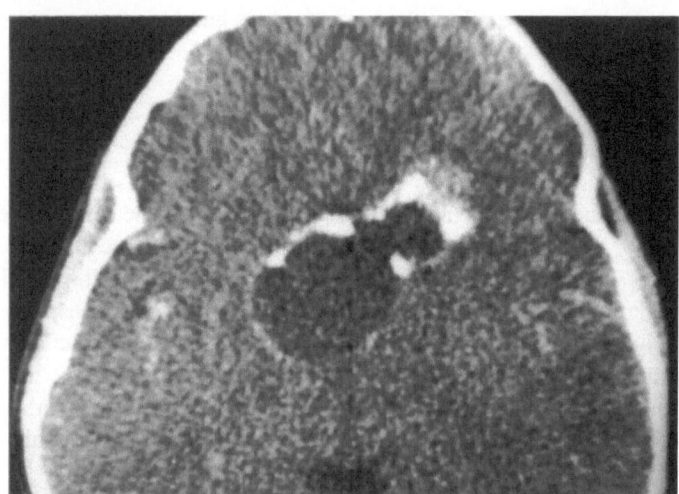

Fig. 1. Axial, nonenhanced CT scan of an 11-year-old boy with visual loss. A complex cystic and partially calcified tumor is demonstrated

moval. In the first 5 years of this study, only 38% of tumors were totally removed, while in the later years of this study primary removal rises to 83% (Table 3). One can note from the data in Table 3 that the number of patients who were undergoing secondary operative procedures has increased in recent years.

Secondary operations were carried out in 34 patients who were operated initially elsewhere. Tumor was removed completly in 47% of this group

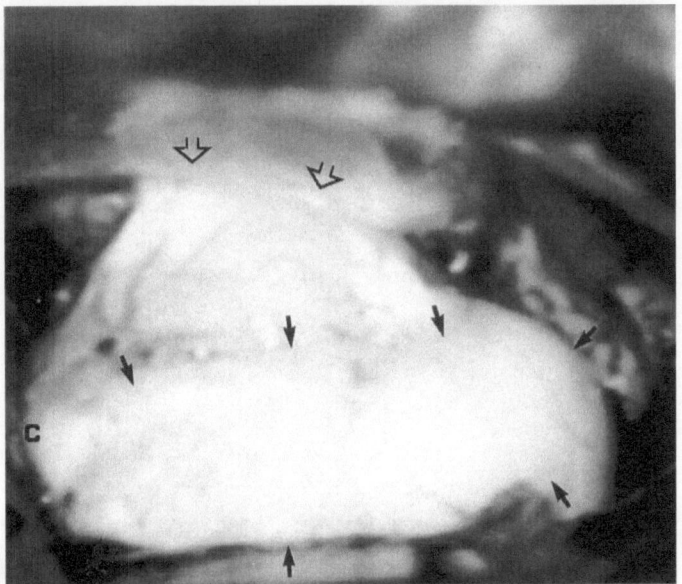

Fig. 2. Operative photograph of right optic nerve in same patient as in Fig. 1. The right optic nerve is seen emerging from the optic foramen (*open arrows*). The chiasm is seen on the left of this view (*C*). A densely calcified white mass is outlined by the *small closed arrows*. No blood vessels are seen in this whitened area, but it appeared to be densely adherent and not separable from the nerve. The child still had vision in the nasal portion of the right visual field

Table 2. Primary operations

Patients	(n)	(%)
Total	65	
• Children	47	
• Adults	18	
Removal total	45	69
• Children	34	72
• Adults	11	61

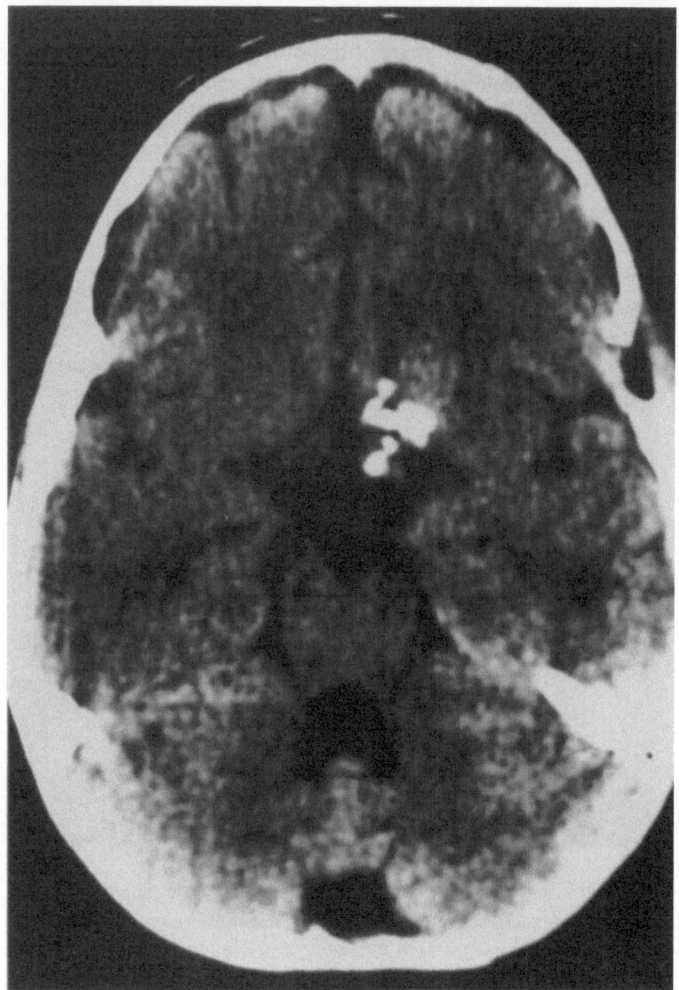

Fig. 3. Postoperative axial CT scan showing the calcifications that remained following removal of the majority of the tumor. This residual tumor was followed carefully
by serial scans. On a contrast-enhanced MRI image approximately 4 years after this
scan was taken, definite soft-tissue growth was noted which had not been present
earlier. At this point the boy was 15 years of age and X-ray therapy was given

(Table 4). However, secondary operations after an initial operative attempt
by the author resulted in two-thirds of these patients being rendered tumor
free. This higher percentage reflects that in a number of these patients the
operator felt that the tumor was totally removed, only to be shown to be
wrong on postoperative CT or magnetic resonance imaging (MRI) scanning.
These "inadvertent" tumor remnants were removed with greater facility.

Secondary Operations

The following two cases illustrate that reoperation after initial operative intervention, radiation therapy (including high intensity radiation therapy), or both does not preclude total tumor removal.

In one patient there was a large cystic tumor with calcification at the base (Fig. 4). An initial operation had been carried out elsewhere at age 6. A radical removal was attempted and the patient was blind in the right eye postoperatively. The tumor recurred within a year and she was reoperated. The surgeon placed a catheter in the tumor bed of the subtotally removed tumor to allow cyst drainage. This is a maneuver that virtually never succeeds because the expanding tumor excludes the catheter as the capsule reforms. (Direct insertion into a virtually intact tumor cavity is required to drain a cystic tumor with a catheter.) At the age of 8 the tumor recurred (Fig. 5) and there was further loss of vision in the remaining left nasal visual field. The patient was referred to the Neurological Institute and radical removal was accomplished at operation (Fig. 6). Two years later the child had 20/40 vision in the left eye and was attending regular school.

Table 3. Total removals

Years	Total patients (n)	Primary operation (n)	Total removal/ primary operation	
			(n)	(%)
1971-1975	13	8	3	38
1976-1980	17	13	8	62
1981-1985	27	20	14	70
1986-1991	42	24	20	83

Table 4. Secondary operations

Patients	(n)	(%)
Secondary operation, primary elsewhere	34	
• Tumor free	16	47
Secondary operation, primary at NINY	15	
• Tumor free	10	67
Three operations at NINY	3	
• Tumor free	1	33
More operations at NINY	2	
• Tumor free	0	

NINY, Neurological Institute of New York

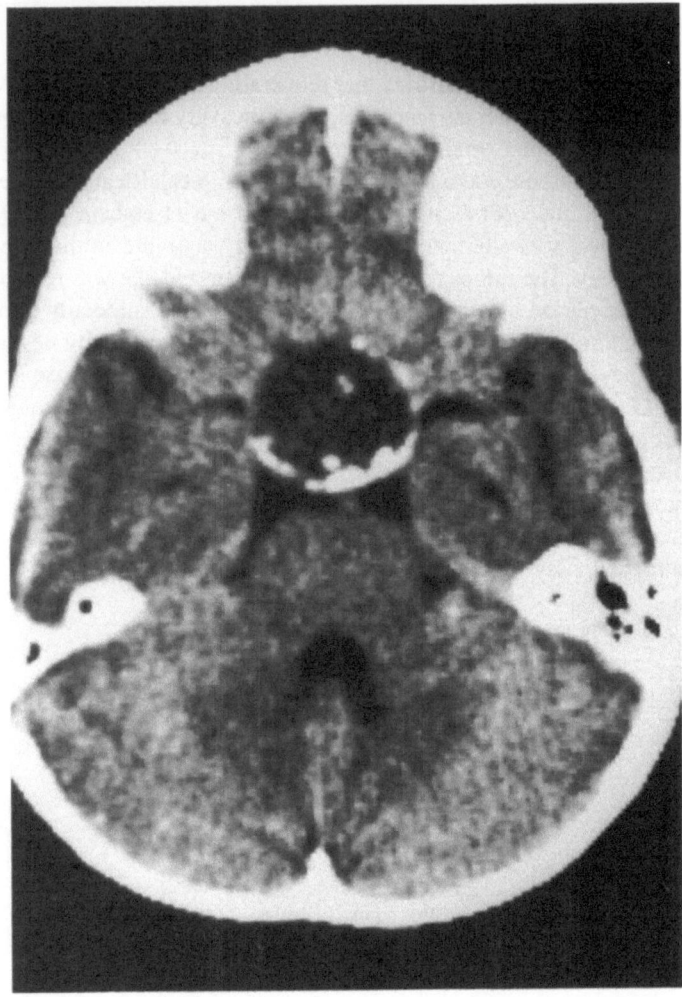

Fig. 4. Axial CT scan of a 6-year-old girl with bitemporal hemianopia. There is a large cystic tumor in the midline. Dense calcifications are noted posteriorly on this scan and dense basal calcifications were noted on lower cuts. An attempt was made to radically remove this tumor at another institution, and postoperatively the child was blind in the right eye with vision only in the nasal field but good acuity in the left eye

The second patient is a 31-year-old woman. She presented initially with signs and symptoms of hydrocephalus. A partially cystic tumor filled the third ventricle (Fig. 7). A shunt was performed in another institution but the patient refused direct operative intervention. She was referred for proton-beam irradiation which was carried out the following year. Eleven months

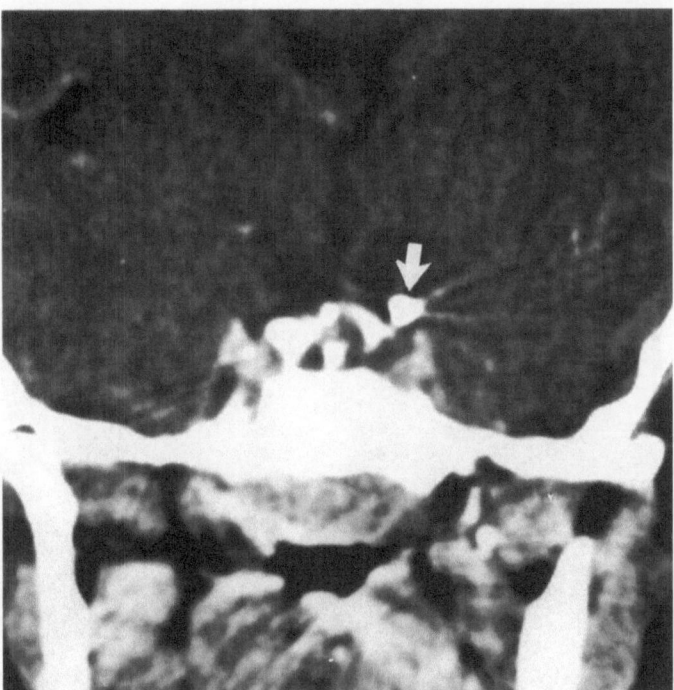

Fig. 5. CT scan taken at the age of 8 of the same child as in Fig. 4. The tumor has recurred and fills most of the sella. Vision is restricted to the inferior nasal quadrant on the left. The radiopaque tip of the catheter intended to drain the tumor cyst is shown at the *arrow*. The catheter has become excluded from the cyst. At operation the catheter indented the under surface of the optic nerve as it joined the chiasm

after the completion of proton-beam irradiation she noted the onset of amenorrhea, headaches, and decreased vision. When she was seen in consultation at the Neurological Institute she had a marked bitemporal hemianopsia and ptosis of the right eye and was lethargic. MRI scan showed good control of hydrocephalus but an increased size of the mass (Fig. 8). The tumor had apparently undergone some cystic degeneration. This tumor was operated on and was totally removed. The pathological examination of the tumor showed that many of the tumor cells had a "mummified appearance." However, areas of apparently viable craniopharyngioma cells still existed (Fig. 9).

Inadvertent Residual Tumor

The next case illustrates the point that tumor tissue inadvertently left after the operator has felt he has accomplished a total removal can often be removed easily at further surgery. In this case a 9-year-old boy with a mostly solid tumor (Fig. 10) was operated on and a "total" removal of felt to be achieved. However, the immediate postoperative CT scan showed a small fragment of residual soft-tissue tumor (Fig. 11). Five days later the child was

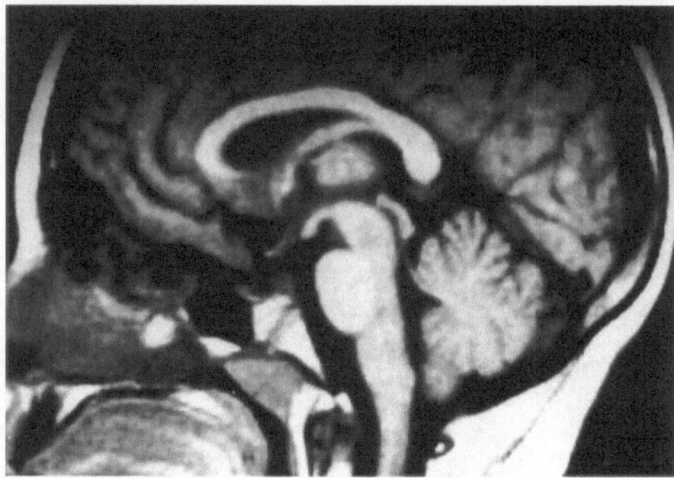

Fig. 6. Postoperative MRI of the same child seen in Figs. 4 and 5. At operation the catheter and the tumor were both removed. Postoperatively she regained the vision in her left nasal field and follow-up acuity at 2 years was 20/40

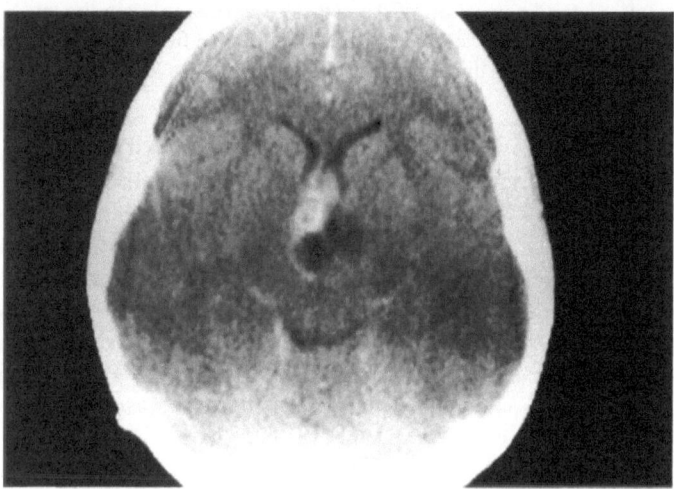

Fig. 7. Axial contrast-enhanced scan in a 30-year-old woman who presented with signs and symptoms of hydrocephalus. The hydrocephalus was controlled by a shunting procedure, but the woman refused direct operative intervention for treatment of her tumor, and she chose to have proton bean irradiation

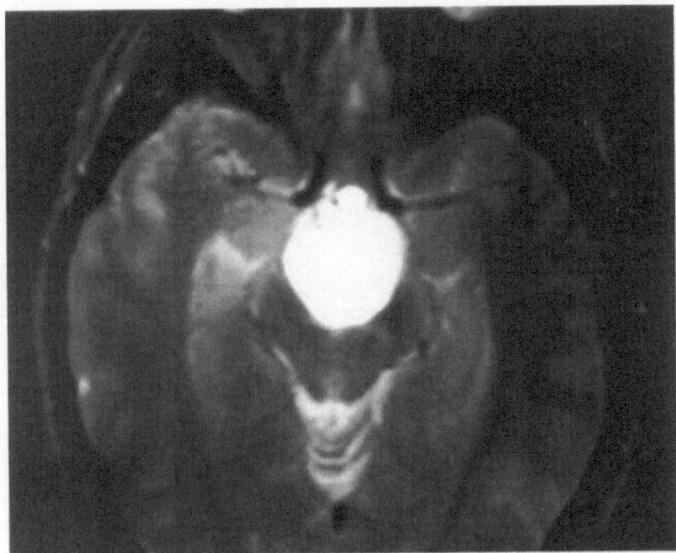

Fig. 8. Axial T2-weighted MRI scan of the same patient as Fig. 7 taken 11 months after proton-beam irradiation. The patient had recently become amenorrheic and complained of headache and decreased vision. There has been a considerable increase in the volume of the tumor when compared to the prior scans and to an immediate postirradiation MRI. The tumor has apparently undergone cystic degeneration

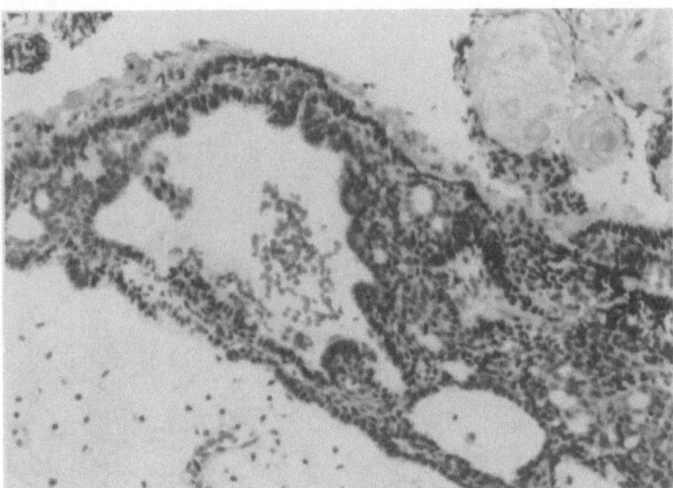

Fig. 9. Pathological specimen of the tumor that was grossly totally removed at operation of patient shown in Figs. 7 and 8. Parts of the tumor specimen showed cells that had a "mummified" appearance. However, the cells in this area of the tumor look entirely viable, with the usual appearance of a craniopharyngioma. A keratinized area of the tumor is shown in the *upper right hand corner*

returned to the operating room. The tumor was not seen initially, but after opening up the lamina terminalis the fragment was found and removed (Fig. 12). In other cases of this type the residual tumor has been followed with

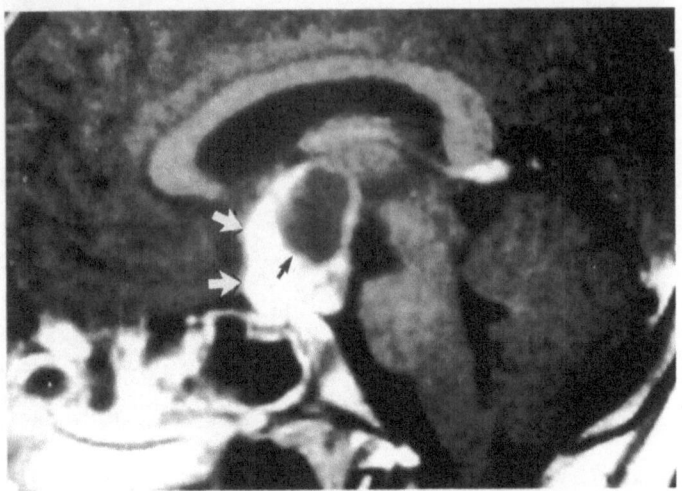

Fig. 10. Sagittal enhanced MRI image of a 9-year-old boy. The tumor is mostly solid with intense contrast enhancement (*white arrows*). The superior portion of the tumor (*black arrow*) was not cystic but rather calcified

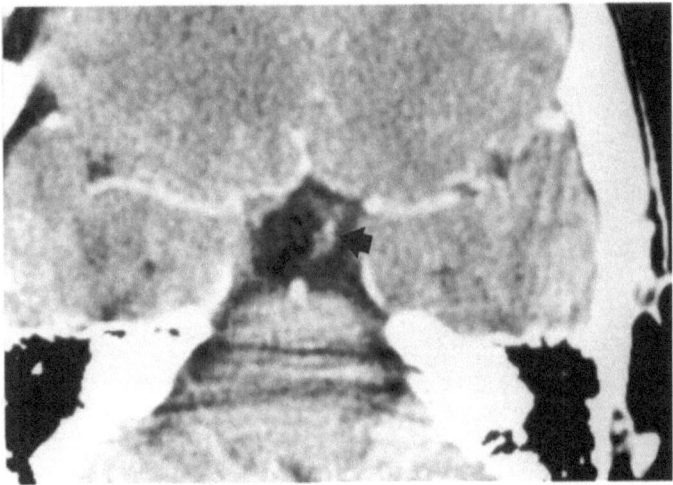

Fig. 11. Contrast-enhanced axial scan taken postoperatively of the same child as shown in Fig. 10. The residual tumor is indicated by the *arrow*. Reoperation was carried out on the fifth postoperative day. The tumor was not seen in the subarachnoid space beneath the chiasm. However, when the lamina terminalis was opened, the fragment was readily identified and removed

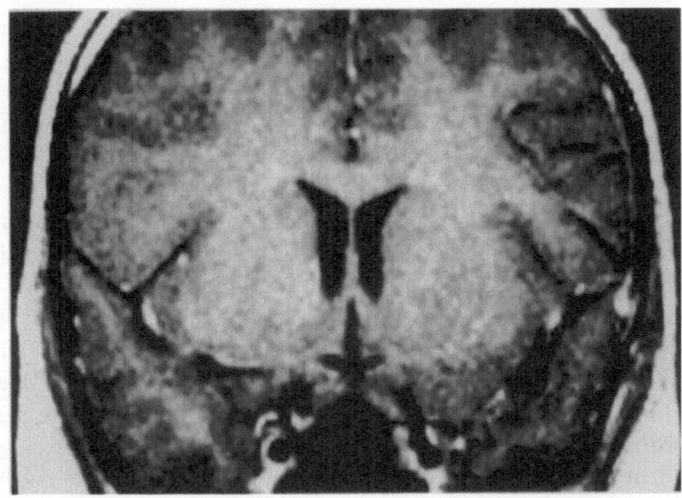

Fig. 12. Coronal, enhanced MRI scan following the second operation on the child shown in Figs. 10 and 11. The fragment has now been removed. The third ventricle has resumed a more normal appearance

serial CT or MRI scans for a number of months, or even several years, until growth of the tumor has been documented, and reoperation has been undertaken at that time.

Preservation of the Pituitary Stalk

In a minority of cases of total removal of the tumor it is possible to spare the pituitary stalk during primary operations (11/72, 15%). The stalk is recognizable first by its constant location in the center of the diaphragm sellae as it leaves the subarachnoid space to enter into the pituitary gland. Second, it is recognizable by its distinctive striate appearance, caused by the long portal veins on the surface of the stalk. These veins retain their parallel appearance no matter how great the distortion of anatomy caused by the bulk of the tumor. After initial debunking of the tumor, it is necessary to enter the suprasellar subarachnoid cistern to find the stalk. The arachnoid is then reflected upward along the stalk in an attempt to keep intact the anastomotic ring of small arteries that supply the median eminence. Often the stalk is found to have quite a good appearance as it penetrates the diaphragm sellae, only to find as the dissection is carried upward to the median eminence that the stalk is progressively thinned out by the tumor and eventually disappears.

Of the 11 patients in whom stalk preservation was possible, three had small intrasellar tumors that were removed via the transsphenoidal approach.

In another patient tumor was removed intracranially and then transsphenoidally. Finally, the pituitary stalk was preserved in seven patients who were operated by craniotomy alone.

Of the 99 patients reported here there was none in whom the pituitary stalk was preserved at secondary operation. However, the following case, operated since 1991, shows that it is possible to preserve the stalk in a secondary procedure. A 32-year-old woman operated at another institution first using a transsphenoidal approach and then transcranial approaches had a tumor with a large cystic component in the suprasellar space and a solid component in the third ventricle (Fig. 13). This tumor was operated transcranially via the subfrontal route and the tumor totally removed. The stalk appears intact in the postoperative MR scan (Fig. 14) and the patient does not require hormonal replacement. Normal menstrual cycles began in the second postoperative month, and she subsequently became pregnant.

In 72 of 99 patients (73%) tumor was removed completely in the course of this work (Table 5); 27 patients are not tumor free (Table 6). Three of the patients with known residual tumor are being followed by CT or MRI scan. Twenty-four have been referred for radiation therapy. Two of these have died of recurrent disease and one has died from causes other than tumor. One patient was moribund during this series and has subsequently died. One patient had a radiation-induced meningioma which suddenly grew over 24 years

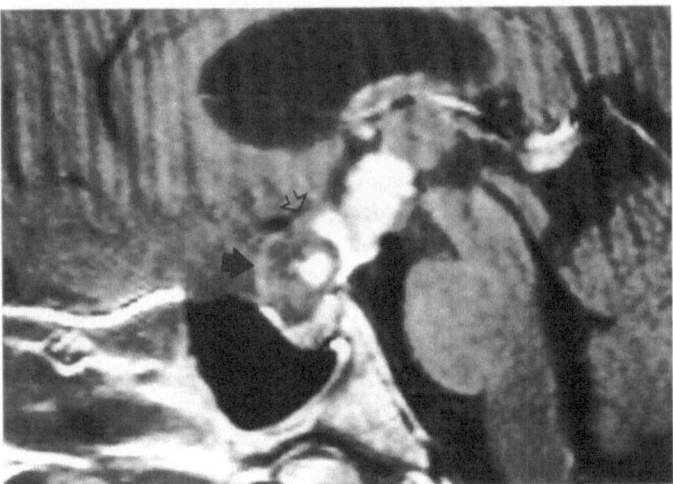

Fig. 13. Sagittal MRI scan after contrast administration of a 32-year-old woman who had undergone prior tumor surgery via transsphenoidal and craniotomy approaches. The cystic portion of the tumor (*solid arrow*) had elevated the chiasm (*open arrow*). The solid, enhancing portion of the tumor lay entirely within the third ventricle. The cystic portion of the tumor was removed subfrontally beneath the chiasm and the lamina terminalis was opened to remove the solid portion of the tumor

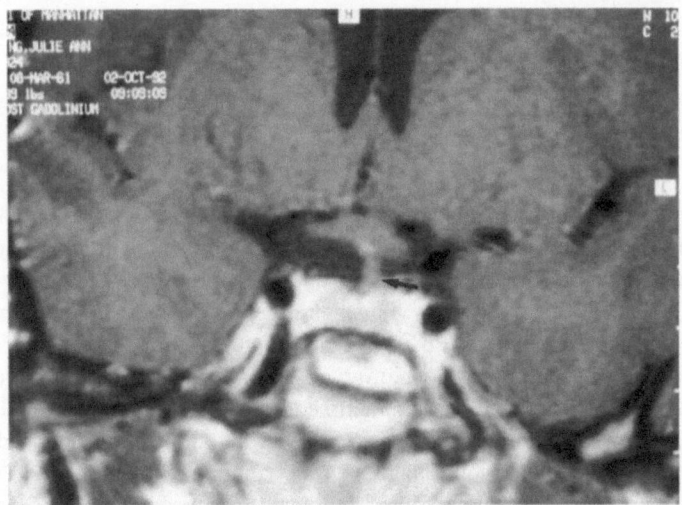

Fig. 14. Postoperative gadolinium-enhanced coronal MRI of the same patient as seen in Fig. 13. The tumor is entirely removed. The pituitary stalk is seen beneath the chiasm and entering the diaphragm sellae. The tumor has left the stalk somewhat deformed and pushed to the left. Enhancement of the upper part of the stalk is normal following contrast injection

Table 5. Tumor-free patients after operation

Patients	(n)
Primary operations	45
Secondary operations [a]	16
Second operation at NINY	10
Third operation at NINY	1
Total	72

NINY, Neurological Institute of New York
[a] Primary operation elsewhere.

Table 6. Non-tumor-free patients after operation

Patients	(n)
Total	27
• Followed up by scan	3
After radiotherapy	24
• Died of intercurrent disease	2
• Died, not due to tumor	1
• Moribund	1
• Secondary radiotherapy-induced tumor	1

after radiation therapy (Fig. 15, B). This tumor was removed but there is a residual portion of the tumor still at the back of the orbit.

Volume Changes

An important factor in adequate management of patients with craniopharyngiomas is consideration of volumes. A 12-year-old boy with a large cystic tumor and massive hydrocephalus was operated upon and a ventricular drain inserted at the time of surgery. Postoperatively, massive subdural hematomas/hygromas developed (Fig. 16). These, in turn, stretched bridging veins and there were multiple venous infarcts. This child had no pressing neurological deficits and there was ample time to treat his hydrocephalus. Had he simply been shunted and allowed to recover, much of the difficulty due to volume displacement would have been prevented. Fortunately, this young boy has made a complete recovery, attends normal school, and has normal vision.

Morbidity and Mortality

Attempts at radical removal at primary operation result in measurable morbidity. Thirteen complications have been noted in ten patients (Table 7). The most serious of these complications are found in three patients with decreased vision in one eye, always on the side of the operative approach. In one patient vision in the other eye was unaffected and in two patients vision improved in the contralateral eye postoperatively.

Morbidity of patients undergoing secondary operations was slightly higher than in the primary operative group (Table 8). In this group there were 51 patients who underwent 68 operations. There were 21 complications occurring in 18 patients. Note that most of these complications were easily treated (e.g., persistent hydrocephalus) or ameliorated with time. The visual deficits produced were entirely limited to the nerve ipsilateral to the side of approach.

There were two deaths due to intercurrent disease. In the first a young boy underwent a "total removal" of his tumor at the age of 8. This tumor extended into the right middle fossa and appeared to be entirely removed. He was operated upon in 1973, before the introduction of CT scanning. The family then moved to Baltimore, Maryland. Three years later a cystic recurrence was found on CT scan in the left side of the posterior fossa. This was subtotally removed in Baltimore. He returned to the emergency room of the Baltimore hospital with acute hydrocephalus and died abruptly.

The second young man was operated in Lebanon at the age of 9. He underwent two craniotomies that year and had conventional radiation therapy.

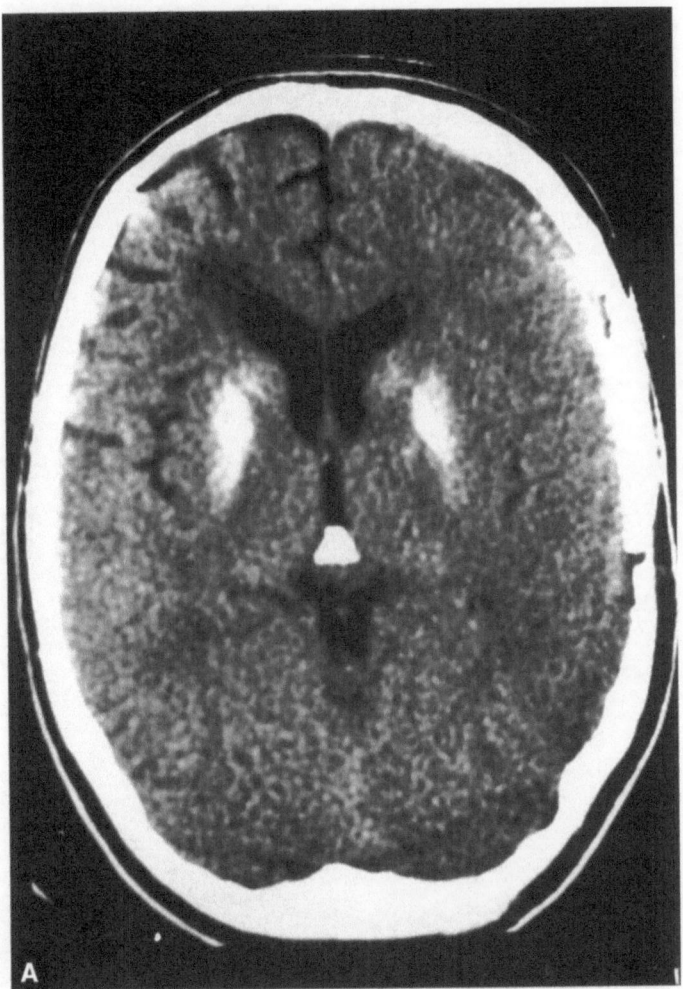

Fig. 15. A Axial CT scan without contrast in a 26-year-old young man who had undergone a subtotal removal of craniopharyngioma at age 4 followed by X-ray therapy. At age 26 he was short in stature, obese and somewhat retarded. The scan showed calcified residual tumor in the suprasellar region which had been unchanged for many years. The calcifications in the basal ganglia and evidence of bifrontal atrophy are common following radiation therapy of the suprasellar region at a young age

At first operation at the Neurological Institute he was 11 years old and subtotal tumor removal was all that could be accomplished, largely because of dense calcification in the suprasellar region extending down the clivus. He was continually troubled by cystic recurrence of tumor in the posterior fossa. Efforts at amelioration, including instillation of ^{32}P isotope into the cysts,

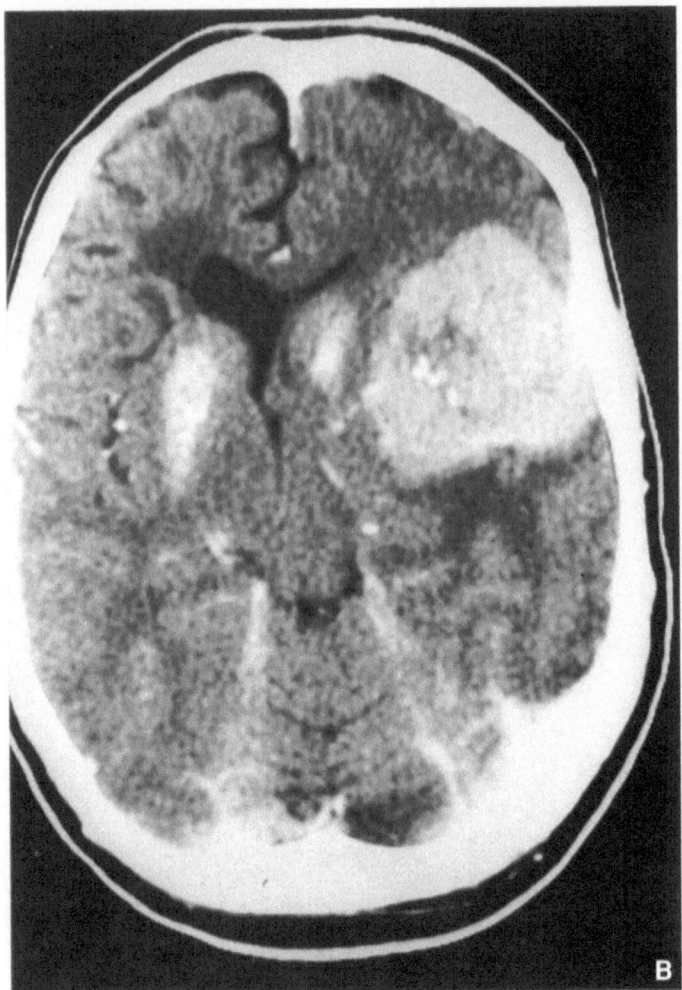

Fig. 15. B Contrast-enhanced axial CT scan of the same patient taken 2 years later. This scan revealed a large sphenoid wing meningioma on the right side. Despite the extremely rapid growth of this tumor, the histological examination indicated a benign meningioma without malignant change. This tumor was totally removed but a recurrence of the tumor in the posterior aspect of the orbit was discovered 2 years later and required another operation. This tumor was in the field of the lateral ports of the X-ray therapy and is a radiation-induced meningioma

were not successful. He underwent a total of six operations and died at the age of 20.

The quality of life in patients in both the tumor-free group and in the non-tumor-free group is quite good. Almost 90% in the tumor-free group are

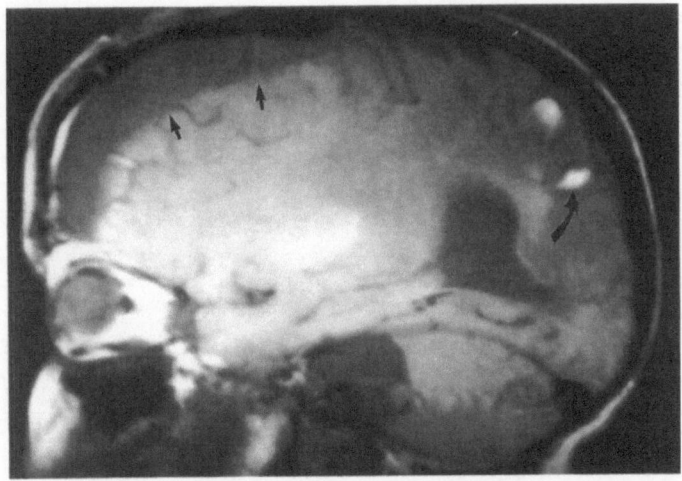

Fig. 16. Postoperative sagittal MRI of a 12-year-old boy with a large cystic tumor and massive hydrocephalus. A ventricular drain was placed at operation and the tumor was removed. Because of the rapid decompression of the cortex, large subdural hygromas (*small arrows*) developed. These hygromas stretched the bridging veins, causing multiple venous infarcts (*large curved arrow*). Fortunately, after a rocky postoperative course, this boy made a complete recovery

either working at a normal job or, if younger, are at their normal school level despite the fact that a significant percentage (10%) have marked visual impairment. Visual impairment remains the most important limiting factor in the postoperative life of these patients.

Discussion

There are three areas in which data derived from this series provide information: (1) total removal, (2) reoperation, and (3) quality of life.

Total Removal

For the greater part of the 20 years covered by this series the goal of operative intervention has been to totally remove the tumor. This goal is by no means accepted by all surgeons. Excellent results have been reported with subtotal removal and irradiation (Baskin and Wilson 1986; Kramer 1976). In addition, others have pointed out that there are serious defects in mentation which may accompany attempts at radical removal (Fisher et al. 1990). A number of recent series have been published which show extremely low

Table 7. Morbidity after 65 primary operations

Complication	n
Decreased vision	3
Cranial nerve deficit	2
Motor deficit	1
Persistent hydrocephalus	4
CSF leak	1
Subdural hygroma	1
Venous infarcts	1
Total complications	12
Patients with complications	10

Table 8. Morbidity after 68 secondary operations

Complication	n
Decreased vision	4
Cranial nerve deficit	2
Motor deficit	2
Hydrocephalus	3
Psychiatric problem	1
Memory deficit	3
Subdural hygroma	1
Flap infection	2
Bone flap removal	1
Distal arterial infarct	1
CSF leak	1
Total complications	21
Patients with complications	15

mortality and acceptable morbidity rates for radical removal (Choux 1991; Hoffman et al. 1992; Laws 1980; Samii and Bini 1991; Symon and Sprich 1985; Yasargil et al. 1990).

It is probably not possible to totally remove all craniopharyngiomas. In addition to the patient with the calcified optic nerve illustrated above, numerous cases are cited in the literature in which a thin cyst wall cannot be removed without leaving small adherent scraps in a number of places. Recent information on instillation of bleomycin into such cysts to thicken the wall and to lessen their growth potential and facilitate their removal have been reported (Broggi et al. 1989; Lapras et al. 1987). Intracavitary instillation of radioisotope for cystic tumors has also been employed successfully (Backlund et al. 1987).

The data from this series indicate that total operative removal can be accomplished in the great majority of patients. Approximately three-quarters of the patients were rendered tumor free. This was accomplished without operative mortality and acceptable morbidity.

The clear benefit of the experience of the surgeon raises a number of important questions. Should these tumors be operated on only at centers where they are commonly seen? If they need to be operated in a noncentralized facility, should a "suboptimal" method of treatment be elected. Polarization of surgeons between conservative and radical modes of therapy makes it unlikely that a multicenter, randomized study will ever be carried out (Sanford and Muhlbaur 1991). The answer may lie in a comparison of the best results of each method.

A number of different operative approaches have been employed in the operations on patients described here. The majority of these were operated on using the right subfrontal approach (Carmel 1985, 1989, 1992; Sweet 1988). In recent years, opening of the lamina terminalis as an adjunct to removal and determination of completeness of resection has been increasingly used (Choux 1991; Lapras et al. 1987). When the tumor is adherent within the third ventricle, an alternative to the lamina terminalis approach can be an approach through the corpus callosum (Yasargil et al. 1990). Intrasellar tumor or those with only a small suprasellar component clearly are best operated using the transsphenoidal approach (Laws 1980). Approach through the temporal fossa has been advocated for those tumors which have a sizable retrosellar component (Symon and Sprich 1985). Finally, a bifrontal approach can be useful, enabling the surgeon to work laterally to both of the optic nerves and tracts (Samii and Bini 1991). The author believes that each of these approaches is useful and may be employed when the occasion demands. The choice of approach is not as important as the determination to surgically remove the tumor completely, if conditions so permit. Surgeons who believe that total removal is not feasible are not likely to achieve it (Hoffman et al. 1992).

Recurrences

Even those surgeons who have taken an aggressive approach to the primary removal of tumors have stressed the difficulty and great risk in reoperation for recurrence (Sweet 1988; Symon and Sprich 1985; Yasargil et al. 1990). Results of this series of patients does not support that notion. While the morbidity for reoperation is somewhat higher than that for primary operations, this increase is not prohibitive. The likelihood of achieving a total removal is also lower with reoperation for tumor recurrence than it is for primary tumors. The exception to this are those cases in which a tumor fragment has been inadvertently left behind, and in such cases the chance of total removal on reoperation is quite good.

Neither prior operation nor irradiation prohibited the successful removal of tumors at a secondary operation. Reoperation should be considered as a useful tool in management of these tumors. This is particularly the case in young children in whom radiation therapy has increasingly deleterious effects (Carmel 1992).

Quality of Life

Most of the patients in this series are now either working normally or attending school at the appropriate grade level. For the great majority of these patients, life is fairly normal, despite the fact that the majority of patients are hormone replacement dependent and more than 10% have serious visual impairment. Visual impairment was the greatest factor which prevented taking on a normal job or attending a normal school. Endocrine deficiencies were not as significant. In those children in whom a hypothalamic type of obesity developed, both social and physical limitations were prominent.

Many of these patients function at an extremely high level. Two are physicians. One boy, operated at the age of 13, now practices pediatric endocrinology at a major midwestern university in the United States. The other, operated in adult years, specializes in internal medicine. Current surgical techniques allow for functional life experiences that are at least as good as those reported with subtotal removal and irradiation. These patients are spared the late effects of radiation therapy and almost three-quarters of them are cured.

The principles derived from this series may contribute to the on-going debate as to the optimum therapy for these most difficult of tumors.

References

Backlund EO, Axelsson B, Bergstrand CG et al (1989) Treatment of cranio-pharyngiomas - the stereotactic approach in a ten to twenty-three year's perspective. I. Surgical, radiological and ophthalmological aspects. Acta Neurochir (Wien) 99:111-118

Baskin DS, Wilson CB (1986) Surgical management of craniopharyngiomas: review of 74 cases. J Neurosurg 65:22

Broggi G, Giorgi C, Franzini A et al (1989) Preliminary results of intracavitary treatment of craniopharyngioma with bleomycin. J Neurosurg Sci 33:45-148

Carmel PW (1985) Tumours of the third ventricle. Acta Neurochir (Wien) 75:136

Carmel PW (1989) Tumors of disordered embryogenesis. In: Youmans JR (ed) Neurological surgery, vol 5, 3rd edn. Saunders, Philadelphia, p 3223

Carmel PW (1992) Transcranial approaches for craniopharyngiomas. In: Apuzzo M (ed) Brain surgery, complications, avoidance and management, part II. Churchill and Livingston, New York (Neoplastic disorders, craniopharyngioma), pp 339-357

Choux M (1991) Craniopharyngioma surgery: techniques, complications and alternatives. Presented at the 59th Annual Meeting of the American Association of Neurological Surgery, New Orleans, 20-25 April

Fischer EG, Welch K, Shillito J et al (1990) Craniopharyngiomas in children; long-term effects of conservative surgical procedures combined with radiation therapy. J Neurosurg 73:534

Hoffman HJ, DeSilva M, Humphreys RP et al (1992) Aggressive surgical management of craniopharyngiomas in children. J Neurosurg 76:47-52

Kramer S (1976) Craniopharyngiomas: the best treatment is conservative surgery and postoperative radiation therapy. In: Morley TP (ed) Current controversies in neurosurgery. Saunders, Philadelphia, p 336

Lapras C, Patet JD, Mottolese E et al (1987) Craniopharyngiomas in childhood; analysis of 42 cases. Prog Exp Tumor Res 30:350

Laws ER Jr (1980) Transsphenoidal microsurgery in the management of craniopharyngioma. J Neurosurg 52:661-111

Samii M, Bini W (1991) Surgical treatment of craniopharyngioma. Zentralbl Neurochir 52:17

Sanford RA, Muhlbaur MS (1991) Craniopharyngioma in children. Neurol Clin 9:453-465

Sutton LN, Gusnard D, Bruce DA et al (1991) Fusiform dilatation's of the carotid artery following radical surgery of childhood craniopharyngiomas. J Neurosurg 74:695

Sweet WH (1988) Craniopharyngiomas (with a note on Rathke's cleft cysts). In Schmidek HH, Sweet WH (ed) Operative neurosurgical techniques. Grune and Stratton, Orlando, p 349

Symon L, Sprich W (1985) Radical excision of craniopharyngiomas. Results in 20 patients. J Neurosurg 62:174

Yasargil MG, Curcic M, Kis M et al (1990) Total removal of craniopharyngiomas: approaches and long-term results in 144 patients. J Neurosurg 73:3

Direct Microsurgery of Craniopharyngiomas: A Review of the Series of the Istituto Neurologico of Milan, Italy

S. Giombini and F. Pluchino

In addressing the problem of craniopharyngioma one is struck by the many-sidedness of the disease, by the controversy that it has always generated, by the successes and, even more, by the unexpected failures of treatment, surgical and other, reported in this battle against an entity often inappropriately termed "benign." Malis' quip about meningiomas of the confluens sinuum "the one good thing about torcular meningiomas is their rarity" (1988) might be applied to craniopharyngiomas but for the unfortunate fact that they are not so rare and thus even this one small virtue is lacking. Wry humor aside, the patient who consults us about a space-occupying lesion of the sellar region that might be a craniopharyngioma always represents a matter to be faced with extreme caution, competence, flexibility, and the heightened awareness that demands total commitment from everyone before, during, and after the surgical act, which of course remains the crucial moment for the future of these patients.

In reviewing the series of the Istituto Neurologico of Milan from the past 12 years, almost entirely the product of the work of the senior author (F.P.), we find proof of the complexity of the problem, due partly to the wide variability of the clinical manifestations, partly to the protean growth of a tumor that produces neuroradiological patterns which are difficult to classify and are very often monstrous and, lastly, to the change that has taken place in surgical philosophy over the years. In the last respect it must be said that our experience reflects that of other large neurosurgical centers round the world; that is, we have moved from a cautious position with the accent on incomplete tumor removal to a more aggressive one aiming at completely radical removal. The rationale underlying this evolution, made possible by the refinement of operating procedures and by the advances in postoperative care, lies in two findings: first, that in achieving a lower rate of recurrence (the chief problem in the follow-up of these patients) the new line has kept the surgical mortality/morbidity rate low; second, the growing conviction that the various therapeutic procedures proposed in the course of the past 20

Division of Neurosurgery, Istituto Nazionale Neurologico "C. Besta", Via Celoria 11, 20133 Milan, Italy

years, interesting though they are, do not provide (or only anecdotally) a permanent solution to the suffering of the craniopharyngioma patient.

The Series of the Istituto Neurologico

Between January 1981 and December 1991 66 patients with craniopharyngioma were referred to our institution and received surgical treatment here. In six of them the lesion was confined to the sella turcica and was an unexpected diagnosis after a transnasosphenoidal operation. The other 60 underwent transcranial microsurgery and constitute the material of this study.

One group of nine patients had been treated elsewhere before admission to our hospital: one patient had received conventional radiotherapy, two gamma knife radiosurgery in Stockholm, and six had been treated surgically, three twice, in every case with incomplete removal.

At the time of their first operation at our institution 17 of the 60 patients were children under 15 years of age (ten boys and seven girls) of mean age 8.9 years and 43 adults (21 men and 22 women) with a mean age of 41.5 years. The distribution by decade of life is given in Fig. 1, which shows peaks in the second, fourth, and fifth decades.

The extrasellar craniopharyngiomas varied enormously in size and extension, both of the solid portion and of the satellite cysts, when present. Only one had developed almost exclusively in the anterior cranial base and clival

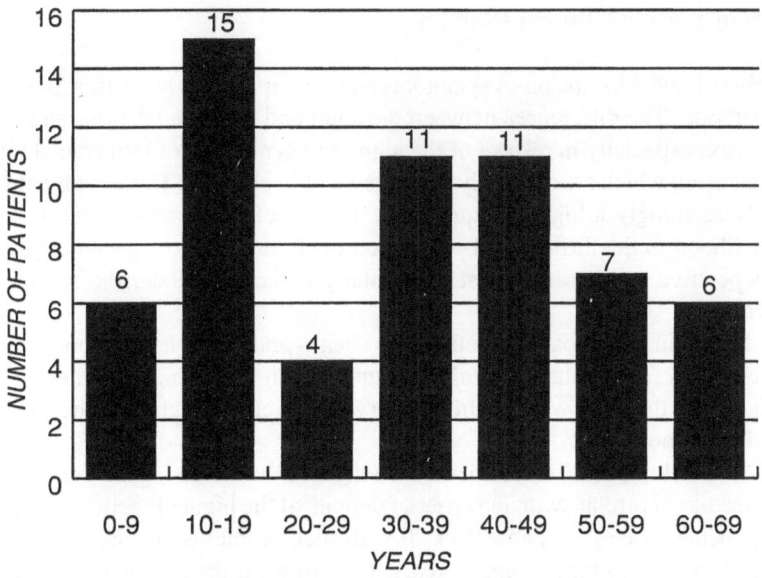

Fig. 1. Age distribution of patients in our series on first observation at our institution

region; of the other 59, 11 were small (< 2 cm) and suprasellar only; all the others exceeded 2 cm at their greatest diameter and in two cases were confined to the third ventricle; in two other cases the development was mainly in a lateral ventricle; in nine cases the tumor involved the anterior, middle, and posterior cranial fossa in various combinations; in the remaining 35 (39%) the site was the most usual one, that is, suprasellar with invasion of the third ventricle.

The exact definition of the site of the craniopharyngioma, of its connections with neighboring structures, especially with the chiasma, and of its solid and cystic components is a key step in the work-up of these patients. To decide on the best surgical strategy the prime requisite is a study in three planes (axial, sagittal, coronal), which only magnetic resonance imaging (MRI) can supply. Since this investigation has been available it has become easier to get a true idea in three dimensions of how the lesion lies and so to plan nonstereotyped and more flexible surgical approaches, often combining several routes in a single operation.

The neuroradiological problems of craniopharyngioma are handled in detail in another section of this book; at this point we wish merely to stress the importance and the difficulty of defining the architecture of craniopharyngioma accurately, that is, of defining it spatially and quantifying the solid and cystic portions. These data do not always fit the operative findings but they are nonetheless of key importance to the planning of surgery.

Preoperative Clinical Pattern

Tables 1 and 2 list the onset symptoms and principal signs at the time of first operation. The differences between the adult and child populations emerge at once, especially in respect of the signs and symptoms of intracranial hypertension which are definitely more frequent in children. There is probably only seemingly a higher frequency of visual defects in adults, due in all likelihood to the difficulty of evaluation in children who as a rule are less cooperative and harder to test, particularly if they are under the age of 2 years.

Endocrine disturbances, both of the adeno- and of the neurohypophysis, are relatively infrequent and often found only in the laboratory. There is a major risk they will worsen after surgery, however, particularly if the aim is radical removal.

As Bartlett (1971) emphasized, the length of the clinical history definitely seems to correlate with the onset of deficits of the higher functions (memory, behavior etc): 14 patients of 20 with such problems, that is, 20%, had had disturbances for less than 2 years. This confirms the finding that mentation disturbances are more often associated with a relatively short history.

Table 1. Initial complaints of children and adults, expressed in percentages

Complaint	Children (%)	Adults (%)
Visual loss	23	35
Headache/vomiting	41	23
Mentation disturbance	6	17
Polyuria	11	9
Short stature	18	–
Amenorrhea	–	9
Loss of libido	–	4
Hypothyroidism	–	2

Table 2. Main clinical findings in children and adults at first admission, expressed in percentages

Clinical finding	Children (%)	Adults (%)
Visual defects (12 blind eyes)	58	95
Papilledema	17	6
Endocrine dysfunction	35	65
Diabetes insipidus	35	30
Psychiatric abnormality	11	41
Hemiparesis	5	2

Surgical Treatment

The 60 patients of our series had surgery once or more than once in which transcranial microsurgical procedures were employed. In 63 of the 71 operations we used the frontotemporal route, extended anteriorly, so that we could make use both of the pterional approach in the strict sense and of the subfrontal approach. In two cases (3%) we used the pterional and transcallosal routes in the same operation and in two other recent cases the interhemispheric route, with sectioning of the anterior communicating artery in order to have access as far as the genu of the corpus callosum and to get an overall view of the extension of the tumor in the third ventricle (Fig. 2). In four patients we used other approaches (anterior transbasal, transcortical for the lateral ventricle, supracerebellar infratentorial, transcallosal), according to the peculiarity of site.

The combination of approaches and the devising of new ones are a somewhat recent development (Arita et al. 1986; Suzuki et al. 1984; Yasargil et al. 1990) which is gathering momentum, partly because of the growing tenden-

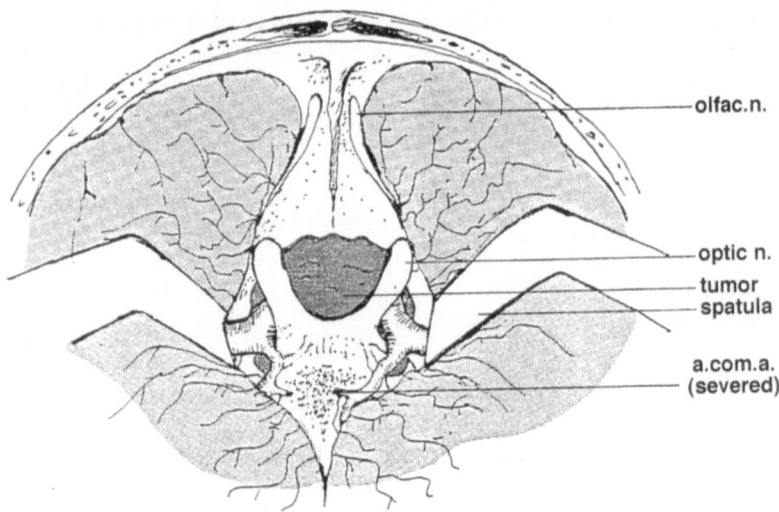

Fig. 2. Interhemispheric approach. Once the bifrontal bone flap has been removed, the superior sagittal sinus is cut basally and the dura is opened bilaterally. Both frontal lobes are retracted and the chiasm is exposed. Both anterior cerebral arteries are isolated: if necessary, the anterior communicating artery (*a. com. a.*) can be severed, widening the exposure of the retrochiasmatic region and the third ventricle. *Olfac. n.* = olfactory nerve

cy towards radical surgery and partly because of the better definition of preoperative imaging which, as mentioned earlier, shows up the advantages and the drawbacks of the various approaches. When making a choice, one also needs to pay attention to the new techniques for operating on the skull base: devised for and tested in other pathological conditions, they can actually be very useful for deep extensions of craniopharyngioma with the aim of avoiding undue retraction of the brain.

Craniotomy for direct attack on the craniopharyngioma was preceded in about half the cases by indirect procedures, which we used from time to time for emergency palliation (aspiration of large cystic components by stereotaxis, performed once or more: 27 cases) or for diagnostic decompressive purposes (gutting via the transnasosphenoidal route: three cases; stereotactic biopsy and radioisotope implantation for brachytherapy: one case), or, lastly, to avert concomitant hydrocephalus when there was doubt about whether the operation would restore patency to the CSF pathways (bilateral ventriculoperitoneal shunting: five cases). In none of the patients did these measures do more than temporarily halt the course of the disease. This point must be kept to the fore in planning the treatment of craniopharyngioma and is a further argument for the greatest possible radicality. The purely cystic variety may be an exception, since the prognosis after intracavitary radioisotope therapy seems to be good (Van Den Berge et al. 1992), at least in respect of tumor growth, but this treatment is not successful in preserving vision or in preventing endocrine deterioration.

Early Surgical Results

For a proper assessment of the results we consider 54 "first direct operations" (direct primary microsurgery) on as many patients who had never undergone craniotomy for craniopharyngioma and 17 reoperations (secondary microsurgery) on 12 patients (six with recurrence after a first operation at our institution and six who came to us after undergoing craniotomy elsewhere).

In the first group there was considerable difference in degree of removal and in operative mortality, depending on the volume (and hence of the supralateroretrosellar extension) of the craniopharyngioma: in 11 cases with a maximum diameter of under 2 cm, complete (gross total) removal was almost the rule and the mortality was zero; in nearly half the patients with larger tumors (25/43, i.e., 58%) removal was incomplete and three patients died (6.9%), two from damage to the hypothalamus and one from intraoperative tearing of the carotid artery.

The overall mortality at first craniotomy in our series was 5.5% (3/54), a figure to be borne in mind when comparing the datum for 17 operations for recurrences. The early morbidity and, even more, the mortality among the latter were more serious: four of the 12 patients died (33%), all due to metabolic disorders arising from diencephalohypophyseal damage, complicated in one case by a DIC. The difference is striking and should be a prime consideration when one has to decide at first operation whether or not to attempt complete removal of the lesion.

Postoperative morbidity also differs markedly, though less, between first operations and reoperations for recurrences (Table 3): ocular status (visual acuity and/or field deficits) worsened in 14% of our patients after the first operation (8/54 operations) and in 35% after reoperation for recurrence (6/17 reoperations). To this must be added the fact that the degree of worsening after reoperation was greater and with less chance of recovery with time. Diabetes insipidus set in in nearly all our patients after first operation and reoperation. This is the inevitable risk of the radical option, which very often results in damage to or abolition of hypothalamohypophyseal function.

Long-Term Surgical Outcome

The mean follow-up of the 53 patients who survived operation was 3.5 years and the range from 1 year in six cases to 11 years after first-operation cases. None was lost to follow-up.

For assessing the long-term outcome (Table 4) we used a Surgical Outcome Scale that takes into account only the patient's clinical status and hence his ability to cope with daily living activities, even in cases in which the neuroradiological follow-up revealed a remnant of craniopharyngioma, as long as it had no tendency to grow. This is the concept of clinical remission used by Baskin and Wilson (1986). The "good outcome" group therefore comprises patients who had undergone radical removal of the lesion, those with incomplete removal but no tumor regrowth, and those with radiologically proven but stable recurrence, that is, all patients who fully resumed their family and social life. Of our 53 patients 42 (14/16 children and 28/37 adults) satisfied this requirement.

The outcome in the remaining 20% (11/53) was fair (1/16 children and 4/37 adults) or poor (1/16 children and 5/37 adults), either because of severe

Table 3. Clinical status shortly after primary and secondary microsurgery

Clinical status	Primary microsurgery (54 procedures)		Secondary microsurgery (17 procedures)	
	(n)	(%)	(n)	(%)
Vision				
• Worsened	8	14	6	35
• Stable	35	64	8	47
• Improved	11	20	3	17
Mentation disturbance	10		3	
Hemiparesis	1		2	

Visual function was evaluated in respect of preoperative condition, taking into account both visual acuity and field defects in each patient.

Table 4. Late surgical outcome of 53 survivors, after a mean follow-up of 3.5 years

Outcome	Children		Adults		Total	
	(n)	%	(n)	%	(n)	%
Good	14	87	28	75	42	80
Fair	1	6	4	11	5	9
Poor	1	6	5	13	6	11

Good, improved, totally independent (clinical remission); fair, some deterioration, moderate psychorganic syndrome, partially dependent; poor, severe deterioration, blindness, major medical problems, totally dependent visual loss (three patients were blind) or serious mental deterioration (five cases) or because of recurrence (two cases) despite more than one reoperation and adjuvant radiosurgery. Only one patient in the "fair" group is disabled because of extraneurological disease, a patient with serious cardiorespiratory disturbances. On analyzing the "poor" outcome group in greater detail, we noted certain features that definitely contributed to poor prognosis: a relatively short clinical history with disorders of the higher functions, large lesion size with voluminous extension within and outside the third ventricle, visual loss and major preoperative endocrine disorders, and more than one operation for recurrence. As one might expect, all these are factors that complicate the management of these patients.

While a more advanced work-up may lead to the earlier discovery of a small craniopharyngioma, the only new and safe way of achieving cure of the disease at first operation and thus avoiding a worse prognosis at later operations is the adoption of a more aggressive and flexible attitude by the neurosurgeon. To this end efforts have been made to devise bolder techniques designed to achieve radical removal at the first craniotomy both by combining approaches in one operation (pterional plus transcallosal, pterional plus interhemispheric, transbasal plus interhemispheric) and by employing unusual approaches for surgery of the intracranial lesions, such as the transbasal route with orbitozygomatic osteotomy or the interhemispheric route with sectioning of the anterior communicating artery.

Peculiarities of the Craniopharyngioma Syndrome

Visual Disturbances

By focusing attention on patients whose chiasmatic syndrome worsened after craniotomy we found that:

1. All had a relatively short clinical history of visual loss (under a year), indicating a tendency to rapid tumor growth.
2. All had large lesions (> 2 cm): four with suprasellar growth only, five extending into the third ventricle, and one extending into the posterior cranial fossa. The cystic component did not predominate, while the solid component was often calcified, making isolation of the capsule from the adjacent neurovascular structures more laborious.
3. In eight cases removal had been subtotal and five of the patients had a recurrence of craniopharyngioma.
4. Of the patients whose postoperative deficit improved, only one had a recurrence that required reoperation.
5. In the group of patients with visual disturbances that worsened after pri-

mary microsurgery, postoperative epileptic seizures and mentation disturbances were more frequent.

By contrast, in the good outcome group the clinical history was less often short, the tumor was not always large, and in the majority of cases removal was radical, with recurrence in only two cases. The inference would seem to be that a large craniopharyngioma and a shorter clinical history carry a higher risk of visual loss, which is frequently associated with cortical dysfunction (epilepsy, slowing) and a higher probability of recurrence.

Endocrine Disturbances

At first examination patients with craniopharyngioma may present few signs and symptoms of endocrine disorder, even if there is massive involvement of the hypothalamohypophyseal region. Only 10% of the patients in our series had symptoms of global or partial hypopituitarism to start with, even though, as others (Thomsett et al. 1980) have observed, more than half showed clinical and laboratory evidence of hormonal disturbance on admission. Diabetes insipidus was present in 31% and stunted growth in 35% (6/17).

All patients had medium grade to severe hypothalamohypophyseal insufficiency immediately after operation, which was uncontrollable in six and ended in their death. Diabetes insipidus developed in 28 cases in addition to the 19 in which it was present preoperatively.

At long-term follow-up there was a slight improvement over the acute postoperative situation, but 49 of the 53 survivors (92.4%) still needed hormone replacement therapy. Only 29 of them had had deficits before operation and so surgery resulted in 20 new cases of hypopituitarism, that is, 38% of the entire series. Diabetes insipidus was still present in 31 of the 53 cases at late follow-up (58.5%), 16 fewer than in the immediate postoperative period but 12 more than before the operation.

These data are in accord with the findings of other authors (Choux et al. 1991; Yasargil et al. 1990) and highlight the extreme importance of hormone replacement in the recovery of patients, whether children or adults, who have had surgery for craniopharyngioma. We can only underline the clear statement of Yasargil, namely, that the strategy of total removal has been made possible by advances in postoperative care.

Recurrences

Recurrence after craniotomy is attributed in the great majority of cases to fragments of the tumor capsule that the surgeon could not or would not remove in order to avoid damage to structures to which it firmly adhered or to remnants of craniopharyngioma missed at operation. Choux et al. (1991) postulate, especially for late recurrences, the development of a new craniopharyngioma from nidi of epithelial cells independent of the radically removed original tumor. The recurrence rate certainly correlates with the type of removal, being higher among cases of incomplete removal (Carmel 1985) (in such cases it would be more appropriate to speak of tumor regrowth), although it is not the rule: Choux et al. (1991) reported a recurrence rate of 63% after subtotal removal versus 25% after total removal. Twenty of our patients had recurrences: five of 27 who had gross total removal (17.3%) and 15 of 30 who had subtotal removal (50%); six of the latter group of patients had had their first operation elsewhere. Twelve were reoperated on by us, seven radically and five subtotally. Two of the latter had a further recurrence and further surgery.

As already emphasized, mortality and morbidity after repeat surgery were high: four deaths, four cases of visual loss, and one case of mental deterioration. The outcome improved slightly with time but at the latest follow-up three patients were in the fair poor group because of major visual and psychic deficits.

Four patients with ascertained recurrences who did not have further surgery received other treatment (radiosurgery in three, brachytherapy in one) for disease progression. Another four were followed up with serial MRI scans, which show that the disease is not progressing, and they will not be offered further treatment as long as the clinical and instrumental status is unchanged.

The difficulty of operating on recurrent craniopharyngioma explains the operative failures, a view shared by the majority of authors (Choux et al. 1991; Konovalov 1981; Yasargil et al. 1990), although Carmel (1985) maintains that the operative risk in recurrences is only "slightly higher." In any case, the decision to reoperate must depend on certain specific parameters: age (radiation therapy, for example, is contraindicated in children under the age of 3), the presence of symptoms (there are cases of instrumental recurrence that remain asymptomatic for a long time), the appearance (cystic and/ or solid) and status (progressing or stable on successive neuroradiological investigations) of the recurrence, and the availability of alternative therapy (gamma knife, LINAC).

Conclusions

On the evidence of the series of the Istituto Neurologico of Milan, Italy, the trend to more aggressive treatment of craniopharyngioma is justified. The high success rate of primary microsurgery and the high failure rate of secondary microsurgery encourage us to redouble our efforts to eradicate the tumor at the first attempt. We thus agree with those who favor total removal (Choux et al. 1991; Hoffman and Raffel 1989; Hoffman et al. 1985; Konovalov 1981, 1987; Matson and Crigler 1969; Sweet 1976; Symon and Sprich 1985; Yasargil et al. 1990), even though a voice as authoritative as that of Baskin and Wilson (1986) affirmed that "subtotal removal followed by radiotherapy is an acceptable treatment for craniopharyngioma." Oddly enough, while theses authors stress the difficulties and risks of radical surgery, they do not consider the far higher risks of reoperation, the illusion that adjuvant radiotherapy is harmless (Amacher 1980; Hoffman and Raffel 1989; Richmond et al. 1980; Ross et al. 1973), and the possibilities now offered by hormone replacement therapy.

With the aid of optimal microsurgical technology in highly skilled hands it will be possible to improve on that 20% of fair/poor outcomes that represents the failure rate in our series and in the largest published series. To achieve this we must act in three directions:

1. Acquire a reliable diagnosis of craniopharyngioma as early as possible, that is, at a stage when the suprasellar development and, hence, damage to the optic pathways and hypothalamus are still reversible.
2. Step up the aggressiveness of craniopharyngioma surgery by means of new strategies tailored to the needs of each patient, with a view to total tumor removal.
3. Foster ever-closer and more imaginative cooperation with the resuscitation staff, endocrinologists, and physiatrists. Such teamwork is essential when one opts for the strategy of total removal, which inevitably involves intricate maneuvers and carries a high risk of neuroendocrine damage, which is most acute and hazardous immediately after operation.

References

Amacher AL (1980) Craniopharyngioma: the controversy regarding radiotherapy. Childs Brain 6:57-64

Arita N, Mori S, Ikeda T, et al (1986) Removal of craniopharyngioma by a unilateral interhemispheric trans-lamina terminalis approach: operative procedures and postoperative management. In: Samii M (ed) Surgery in and around the brain stem and the third ventricle. Springer, Berlin, Heidelberg, New York, pp 389-395

Bartlett JR (1971) Craniopharyngiomas. An analysis of some aspects of symptomatology, radiology and histology. Brain 94:725-732

Baskin DS, Wilson CB (1986) Surgical management of craniopharyngiomas. A review of 74 cases. J Neurosurg 65:22-27

Carmel PW (1985) Craniopharyngiomas. In: Wilkins RH, Rengachary SS (eds) Neurosurgery. McGraw-Hill, New York, pp 905-916

Choux M, Lena G, Genitori L (1991) Le craniopharyngiome de l'enfant. Neurochirurgie 37 (Suppl. 1):1-174

Grant DB, Lyen K (1982) Hypopituitarism after surgery for craniopharyngioma. Childs Brain 9:201-204

Hoffman HJ, Raffel C (1989) Craniopharyngiomas. In: McLaurin RL, Venes JL, Schut L, Epstein F (eds) Pediatric neurosurgery, 2nd edn. Saunders, Philadelphia, pp 399-408

Hoffman HJ, Chuang S, Ehrlich R, et al (1985) The microsurgical removal of craniopharyngiomas in childhood. Conc Pediatr Neurosurg 6: pp 52-62

Konovalov AN (1981) Operative management of craniopharyngiomas. Adv Tech Stand Neurosurg 8:291-318

Konovalov AN (1987) Technique and strategies of direct surgical management of craniopharyngioma. In: Apuzzo MLJ (ed) Surgery of the third ventricle. Williams and Wilkins, Baltimore, pp 542-553

Matson DD, Crigler JF (1969) Management of craniopharyngioma in childhood. J Neurosurg 30:377-390

Richmond IL, Wara WM, Wilson CB (1980) Role of radiation therapy in the management of craniopharyngiomas in children. Neurosurgery 6:513-517

Ross HS, Rosenberg S, Friedman AH (1973) Delayed radiation necrosis of the optic nerve. Am J Ophthalmol 76:683-685

Suzuki J, Katakura R, Mori T (1984) Interhemispheric approach through the lamina terminalis to tumors of the anterior part of the third ventricle. Surg Neurol 22:157-163

Sweet WH (1976) Radical surgical treatment of craniopharyngioma. Clin Neurosurg 23:52-79

Symon L, Sprich W (1985) Radical excision of craniopharyngioma. Results in 20 patients. J Neurosurg 62:174-181

Thomsett MJ, Conte FA, Kaplan SL, et al (1980) Endocrine and neurologic outcome in childhood craniopharyngioma: review of effect of treatment in 42 patients. J Pediatr 97:728-735

Van Den Berge JH, Blaauw G, Breeman WAP, et al (1992) Intracavitary brachytherapy of cystic craniopharyngiomas. J Neurosurg 77:545-550

Yasargil MG, Curcic M, Kis M, et al (1990) Total removal of craniopharyngiomas. Approaches and long-term results in 144 patients. J Neurosurg 73:3-11

Surgical Craniopharyngioma Treatment

V.V. Dolenc, G. Mariniello, A. Horvat, J. Sustersic, B. P. Prestor, and R. Pregelj

Introduction

Craniopharyngiomas are histologically benign tumors of maldevelopmental origin, occurring mainly in the intra- and suprasellar regions. These neoplasms arise from epithelial remnants of squamous cells of Rathke's pouch stomodeal epithelium. Craniopharyngiomas represent 2.5%-3% of all intracranial tumors. About 50% of them occur in childhood. These tumors may be predominantly cystic (with no significant solid portion), mixed (cystic and solid components), or predominantly solid. The fluid in the cysts varies but is usually brownish, containing cholesterol crystals. In all cases craniopharyngiomas have a stratified squamous epithelium resting on a collagenous basement membrane.

According to Yasargil et al. (1987) the location of craniopharyngiomas may be (a) intrasellar-infradiaphragmatic, (b) intra- and suprasellar (infra- and supradiaphragmatic), (c) supradiaphragmatic, parachiasmatic, extraventricular, (d) intra- and extraventricular, (e) paraventricular (mainly extending to the third ventricle), and (f) intraventricular. A retrochiasmatic expansion of a craniopharyngioma into the hypothalamus and/or into the third ventricle is the most difficult, as complete excision mostly affects the hypothalamic functions.

In both children and adults, a craniopharyngioma most frequently causes visual deficits. Endocrine abnormalities and signs and symptoms of increased intracranial pressure due to hydrocephalus occur either alone or follow the visual deterioration. Other focal cerebral deficits are present only occasionally.

The ideal treatment of craniopharyngiomas is total microsurgical excision of the lesion which, in the majority of cases, results in the restoration of neuroendocrinological functions. In patients in whom total excision of the lesion is impossible due to the adhesion of the tumor capsule to the perforating arteries, or due to the extension of the tumor into the hypothalamus, it is

Department of Neurosurgery, University Hospital Center, Zaloska 7
61105 Ljubljana, Slovenia

wiser to retreat so as not to damage the vasculature of the hypothalamus, of the chiasm, of the pituitary stalk and of the optic tracts. In such cases it is advisable to leave the portion of the capsule which is adherent to the hypothalamus, the pituitary stalk, or visual apparatus and to monitor the patient with regular magnetic resonance imaging (MRI). In cases of incomplete resection of the craniopharyngioma, radiotherapy as complementary treatment is recommended by some authors (Backlund 1973, 1987; Kramer 1976), whereas other authors favor complete resection of the lesion (Al-Mefty et al. 1985; Sweet 1976; Symon and Sprich 1986; Yasargil et al. 1990). After increased experience gained from operating on craniopharyngioma cases, the senior author of this paper holds the same view as the latter group of authors.

Under no circumstances do we support radiation therapy in the treatment of patients with craniopharyngiomas because it offers no guarantee that the tumor will stop growing, and furthermore, it will certainly cause scarring and late ischemic lesions of the neighboring vital structures.

Patients

Of 64 patients with craniopharyngioma treated at our department, 42 had previously been operated on in other institutions. Of these 42 patients, 35 had undergone earlier operations for hydrocephalus: ventriculoatrial shunts were inserted in 10 cases and ventriculoperitoneal shunts in 25, and following these procedures, nonmicrosurgical and, in some cases, so-called microsurgical partial resections of the lesions were carried out. Seven of these 42 patients had also been previously treated with radiotherapy after the initial incomplete resection of the lesion, and four had been treated with intracystic yttrium. In all 42 patients, deterioration following initial improvement after a shunting procedure and/or surgical exploration of the tumor was ascribed to the so-called recurrent tumor.

Of the 64 patients of the series, 30 were under 13 years of age, and the remaining 34 were older. Thirty-one patients were female and 33 were male. The leading symptom was visual deterioration, which was found in 47 patients and manifested itself either as a visual field defect or decreased visual acuity. Hypothalamic-hypophyseal disturbances were present in 21 patients. In the group of 22 patients admitted for primary surgery, hydrocephalus was present only in three patients and was solved by complete removal of the tumor so that shunting was not required (Fig. 1). The patients were evaluated with computed tomographic (CT) scanning and/or MRI.

All the operations were carried out by the senior author (V.V.D.). The surgical strategies were planned with regard to the size, shape, location, and consistency of the craniopharyngiomas. In all but three patients, a modified pterional approach was employed (Dolenc 1985; Dolenc et al. 1987, 1994),

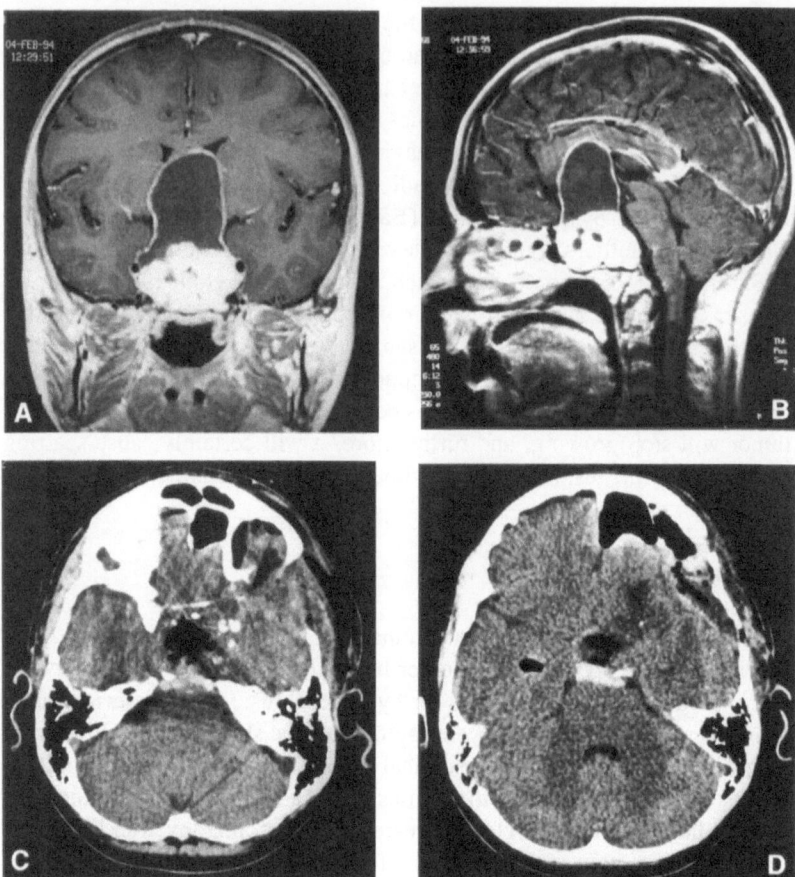

Fig. 1 A-D. Preoperative MRI and postoperative CT scans in a 26-year-old male patient. **A** Coronal and **B** sagittal MRI views showing a partly solid and partly cystic giant craniopharyngioma. The tumor was gross totally removed through the right-sided transorbital-transclinoid-transsellar-transsylvian approach. **C, D** Postoperative axial CT scans showing a small residual tumor. Postoperatively the patient noted improvement of visual acuity while endocrinological disturbances remained the same. He also suffered from hypothalamic dysfunction, i.e., increased appetite (polyphagia) and diabetes insipidus, both of which disappeared within 3 weeks after surgery

and in the remaining three patients a combination of the interhemispheric-transcallosal-transforaminal approach and a modified pterional approach was employed. The transsphenoidal approach was not used because in none of the patients in our series was the lesion confined to the sella alone (Laws 1980). In all but three cases the resection of the tumor was complete. Two patients of the series had recurrence after primary surgery at our department and underwent a second procedure for total excision of the tumor.

Surgical Technique

The patient is positioned in the supine position on the table and the head is rotated to the left and then fixed in a tripoint Mayfield headrest so that the orbitozygomatic junction is the highest point. The cutaneous, the muscular, and the bone flaps are formed as in the cavernous sinus (CS) approach. The orbital roof posterior to the superior orbital fissure (SOF) is removed to the foramen ovale, so that the SOF is completely free. Following this, the sphenoid wing and the anterior clinoid process (ACP) are removed and the optic canal opened on the dorsolateral aspect. Care should be taken not to damage the optic nerve, the third and fourth cranial nerves, or the internal carotid artery (ICA) in the area of the anteromedial triangle (Dolenc 1989). The dural tent connecting the dura of the temporal lobe with the periorbit is cut along the longitudinal axis of the third, fourth, and sixth cranial nerves, and then peeled from these nerves in a centripetal direction. The inner membrane of the lateral wall of the normal CS should be preserved intact in order to prevent venous bleeding from the CS. The next step is an incision into the dura along the sylvian fissure anteriorly toward the dural ring around the ICA. The dural edges are then fixed with stay sutures to the left and to the right. The sylvian fissure is split completely in the usual way, starting from the periphery to the middle cerebral artery (MCA) and then along it down to the bifurcation of the ICA. When the frontal and temporal lobes are completely divided and the whole segment of the MCA exposed, the frontal lobe is slightly retracted and the anterior cerebral artery A1 (ACA1) is followed toward the anterior communicating artery (ACom) and beyond the midline so that the contralateral ACA1 is also visualized. In cases where the tumor is in the sella, i.e., under the diaphragm sellae, the dural ring around the ICA should be cut circumferentially and the initial segment of the ophthalmic artery exposed coursing from the ICA into the optic canal. When the dural ring is cut round-and-round the ICA and the anterior loop of the ICA is freed, the tumor is removed from the sella through the approach behind the anterior loop of the ICA, i.e., lateral to the intradural ICA and anterior to the posterior clinoid process (PCP). Accidental venous bleeding from the ipsilateral CS can easily be stopped by packing the CS with Surgicel, but not too tightly or the intracavernous segment of the ICA will be compressed. If the craniopharyngioma extends downward along the clivus, the PCP is resected by drilling it off from the intrasellar side toward the dura posteriorly. The dorsum sellae together with the PCP is removed down to the floor of the sella. This allows exposure of the retrosellar segment otherwise hidden behind the dorsum sellae. At the same time, the removal of the PCP also enables the surgeon to reach the bifurcation of the basilar artery and to remove the tumor from the upper brainstem and along both P1s and both posterior communicating arteries (PCom), as well as from both oculomotor nerves.

The space gained with the removal of the ACP and PCP allows the surgeon to work in an upward direction along the pituitary stalk and in the area of the hypothalamus. All the perforating arteries originating from the circle of Willis as well as those (Dawson's arteries) originating from the ICA and running toward the chiasm, the pituitary stalk, and the optic tracts should be preserved intact. It is therefore wiser to debulk the tumor from the inferolateral aspect of the intradural ICA rather than through the space between the optic nerve and the ICA or from above, entering inbetween both optic nerves and anterior to the chiasm. Only when the tumor is sufficiently debulked from below can the rest of the mass be removed through the upper two apertures, i.e., through the gap between the optic nerve and the ICA and through the space between both optic nerves. During removal of the tumor, no traction should be exerted so as not to damage the perforating arteries or veins. Irrigation with saline should be sufficient to prevent drying out of these vessels, the ICA, and the visual apparatus.

In most cases the craniopharyngioma can be removed as described. Only in the cases in which the tumor extends into the hypothalamus or into the third ventricle should the interhemispheric-transcallosal-transforaminal approach be used and the tumor debulked (Apuzzo et al. 1982, 1987), while the rest of the tumor is removed as described earlier in the text (Konovalov 1987; Yasargil et al. 1987). It is not only difficult but also risky to remove a craniopharyngioma in this location using exclusively the interhemispheric-transcallosal-transforaminal approach. For this reason, a combination of both approaches is necessary (Yasargil et al. 1987).

The described transorbital-transclinoid-transsylvian approach provides the surgeon with sufficient working space so that the whole lesion can be removed without retracting the brain and without working in hidden corners behind the structures, in which case bleeding might occur.

Discussion

Craniopharyngiomas are most often located in the central skull base, i.e., in the sella and in the parasellar area, and may spread into the visual apparatus, the circle of Willis, the perforating arteries from the circle of Willis, and in some cases the hypothalamus and even the intraventricular and/or intracerebral space. Since craniopharyngiomas are not only expansive but may also be infiltrative, they affect the pituitary, hypothalamic, and visual functions. With further extension or infiltration the tumor may also damage the functions of the more distant structures, i.e., the frontal lobes, medial portions of the temporal lobes, striocapsulothalamic areas, mamillary bodies, and limbic system. As the tumor progresses into the third ventricle and occludes one or both of the foramina of Monro, unilateral or bilateral hydrocephalus will occur.

The treatment of choice for a craniopharyngioma is complete resection of the lesion without any surgery-related morphological and/or functional lesion of the surrounding structures (Baskin and Wilson 1986; Konovalov 1981; Patterson and Danylevich 1980; Symon and Sprich 1985; Yasargil et al. 1987, 1990). However, even the most skilled hands employing the most meticulous microsurgical techniques cannot, in some large craniopharyngiomas, cope with the extremely difficult or even impossible dissection of the normal structures from the tumor (Bucci et al. 1987; Rougerie 1979). In such cases the surgeon is faced with a difficult dilemma, i.e., proceed with resection of the lesion which will inevitably damage the normal surrounding tissue or retreat and treat the rest of the tumor with complementary modalities (Richmond et al. 1980). At this point it is difficult to make the right decision, especially for someone who has insufficient experience. The surgeon can make the mistake of going too far with the resection of the capsule of the craniopharyngioma and thereby create extremely difficult and long lasting, if not permanent, endocrinological deficits. Another possible "mistake" that can be made (and is in fact often made) is partial resection of the craniopharyngioma (debulking), which results in a good postoperative outcome: visual function may improve, the endocrinological functions remain the same, and hydrocephalus can be dealt with by an additional shunting procedure. To these "clever and cautious procedures," other dangerous procedures may be added, i.e., instillation of yttrium or other radiotherapy. However, all these procedures in combination only serve to prolong the period of so-called "ill-health" tolerance which will ultimately lead to more severe, if not unsolvable, problems. The protagonists of this multimodality treatment for craniopharyngiomas are still in the majority, and it will take a long time before it is generally accepted that primary surgical treatment, which should provide complete excision of the lesion, is the treatment of choice for craniopharyngiomas.

It is also true that patients with craniopharyngiomas, especially those with major disturbances of endocrinological equilibrium in whom the metabolism of water and electrolytes is in question (hypothalamic dysfunction), should be treated surgically and medically (postoperatively) in centers where team work can be provided. Team work in the treatment of craniopharyngiomas afflicting the function of the hypothalamus is mandatory since there is no way to forecast the endocrinological imbalance and changes in the metabolism of water and electrolytes either after partial and even less after complete resection of the lesion.

In all our patients operated on primarily, even in those with preexisting hydrocephalus, the shunt was not used since it was believed that removal of the tumor would regulate the circulation of the CSF, which in fact was the case.

In addition to hydrocephalus, the rapid loss of vision also calls for emergency removal of the tumor. The compression by the tumor from the lower aspect against the chiasm, optic nerves, and optic tracts, in combination with the strangulation by the overlying and stretched ACA1s, can cause rapid loss of vision unilaterally or even bilaterally. Careful and complete removal of the lesion can preserve the remaining vision, or even improve it.

Cases of endocrinological disturbances are the least urgent and there is always enough time to obtain a second opinion. It is also true that very slight endocrinological disturbances may become an unsurmountable problem after surgery.

Complete excision of the craniopharyngioma was carried out in all cases of primary surgery in our series and endocrinological deficits either did not occur or were only of a transient character. In 80% of patients with preoperative visual deterioration, visual function improved after surgery. In 15% the visual deficits remained the same, and in 5% they were aggravated. In craniopharyngiomas causing hydrocephalus, complete removal of the lesion reestablished normal CSF circulation. In the series of secondary surgery patients, complete resection was achieved in 90% and in 10% subtotal resection of the lesion was possible. In patients in whom changes due to radiotherapy or previous surgery caused scarring of the peripheral parts of the craniopharyngioma and thence adhesions to the normal tissue, complete removal of the tumor was considered too risky, i.e., the probability of creating permanent lesion of the visual apparatus, hypothalamus, and/or third and fourth cranial nerves was very great. As a result of our experience we hold that partial excision of the craniopharyngioma combined with radiotherapy and/or instillation of yttrium should in no case be the first consideration. We favor primary surgery in which, whenever possible, the tumor is completely removed. It is also advisable that craniopharyngiomas, when large and causing a lesion of the pituitary stalk and/or hypothalamus, should be treated in well-equipped centers where appropriate teams are available and where sufficient experience (surgical and medical) has been gained through the frequent treatment of such cases. We also believe that the real emergency in craniopharyngioma is hydrocephalus and a rapid deterioration of vision which can only temporarily be solved by shunting.

The transorbital-transclinoid-transsellar-transsylvian approach enables an experienced neurosurgeon to completely resect the craniopharyngioma without any retraction of the brain or other neural structures. By using an appropriate approach and appropriate microtechniques, the complete removal of a craniopharyngioma at primary surgery should not be a problem in most cases. And in patients in whom complete resection of the lesion is too risky, even in highly skilled hands, it is wise to leave the adherent part of the capsule of the tumor alone and to monitor the patient rather than to treat him with radiation. In most cases, additional surgical treatment of a recurrent tumor will be much less devastating than radiotherapy. Radiotherapy or gamma knife surgery might prove useful only if surgery fails.

References

Al-Mefty 0, Hassaounah M, Weaver P (1985) Microsurgery for giant craniopharyngiomas in children. Neurosurgery 17:585-595

Apuzzo MLJ, Chikovani OK, Gott PS (1982) Transcallosal, interfornicial approaches for lesions affecting the third ventricle: surgical considerations and consequences. Neurosurgery 10:547-554

Apuzzo MLJ, Zee C, Breeze RE (1987) Anterior and mid-third ventricular lesions: a surgical overview. In: Apuzzo MLJ (ed) Surgery of the third ventricle. Williams and Wilkins, Baltimore, pp 518-520

Backlund EO (1973) Studies on craniopharyngiomas. III. Stereotaxic treatment with intracystic yttrium-90. Acta Chir Scand 139:237-247

Backlund EO (1987) Role of stereotaxis in the management of midline cerebral lesions. In: Apuzzo MLJ (ed) Surgery of the third ventricle. Williams and Wilkins, Baltimore, pp 802-805

Baskin DS, Wilson CB (1986) Surgical management of craniopharyngiomas. A review of 74 cases. J Neurosurg 65:22-27

Bucci MN, Chin LS, Hoff JT (1987) Perioperative morbidity associated with operative resection of craniopharyngioma: a review of ten years experience. Neurochirurgia 30:135-138

Dolenc VV (1985) A combined epi- and subdural direct approach to carotid-ophthalmic artery aneurysms. J Neurosurg 62:667-672

Dolenc VV (1989) Anatomy and surgery of the cavernous sinus. Springer, Berlin Heidelberg New York

Dolenc VV, Skrap M, Sustersic J, Skrbec M, Morina A (1987) A trancavernous-transsellar approach to the basilar tip aneurysms. BJN 1:251-259

Dolenc VV, Prestor BP, Sustersic J, Pregelj R (1994) Transclinoid-transsellar-transcavernous approach to basilar tip aneurysms. In: Pasqualin A, Da Pian R (eds) New trends in management of cerebro-vascular malformations. Springer, Vienna, pp 231-237

Konovalov AN (1981) Operative management of craniopharyngiomas. Adv Tech Stand Neurosurg 8:291-318

Konovalov AN (1987) Technique and strategies of direct surgical management of craniopharyngioma. In: Apuzzo MLJ (ed) Surgery of the third ventricle. Williams and Wilkins, Baltimore, pp 542-553

Kramer S (1976) Craniopharyngioma: the best treatment is conservative surgery and postoperative radiation therapy. In: Morley TP (ed) Current controversies in neurosurgery. Saunders, Philadelphia, pp 336-343

Laws ER (1980) Transsphenoidal microsurgery in the management of craniopharyngiomas. J Neurosurg 52:661-666

Patterson RH, Danylevich A (1980) Surgical removal of craniopharyngiomas by a transcranial approach through the lamina terminalis and sphenoid sinus. Neurosurgery 7:111-117

Richmond IL, Wara WM, Wilson CB (1980) Role of radiation therapy in the management of craniopharyngiomas in children Neurosurgery 6:513-517

Rougerie J (1979) What we can expect from the surgical treatment of craniopharyngiomas in children. Report of 92 cases. Childs Brain 5:433-449

Sweet WH (1979) Recurrent craniopharyngiomas: therapeutic alternatives. Clin Neurosurg 27:206-229

Symon L, Sprich W (1985) Radical excision of craniopharyngiomas. Results in 20 patients. J Neurosurg 62:174-181

Yasargil MG, Teddy PJ, Roth P (1987) Combined approaches. In: Apuzzo MLJ (ed) Surgery of the third ventricle. Williams and Wilkins, Baltimore, pp 462-475

Yasargil MG, Curcic M, Kis M (1990) Total removal of craniopharyngiomas. Approaches and long-term results in 144 patients. J Neurosurg 73:3-11

Surgical Management of Craniopharyngiomas from 1976 to 1992: Problems and Results

R. M. VILLANI*, E. P. SGANZERLA*, S. M. GAINI*, L. BELLO*, AND M. GIOVANELLI

Introduction

Although Northfield's opinion of 1957 that: "the treatment of these (cranio-pharyngioma) patients is fraught with difficulty and disappointment to a degree probably not offered by any other intracranial tumor with exception of glioblastoma" nowadays sounds unacceptably pessimistic, craniopharyngioma surgery is still a major challenge, even for experienced neurosurgeons, and many consider it one of the most delicate intracranial procedures (Baskin and Wilson 1986; Cushing 1932; Hoffman et al. 1992; Katz 1975; Manaka et al. 1985). Some of the major obstacles to achieving the desired therapeutic goal, i.e., total tumor removal without unacceptable functional deterioration of the patient, are:

- The critical location of these histologically benign tumors in the sellar/ parasellar area with the firm attachments which may intervene between the epithelial neoplastic cells and the pituitary stalk, the hypothalamus, the visual pathways, and the arteries of the anterior part of the circle of Willis
- The direct involvement of vital brain areas possibly associated with manifold functional disorders, the most common of which are visual dysfunction, diabetes insipidus, various degrees of endocrine failure, disturbances of heat regulation, vasomotor disturbances, sleep disorders, and emotional changes
- The sometimes very large tumor volumes with villous elongations extending to surrounding brain and ventricular cavities.

Complete tumor removal was already advocated by Matson (1969), Matson et al. (1969), and Sweet (1976), who described that in most cases a cleavage plane between the tumor capsule and the vitally important brain structures can indeed be found and nervous structures preserved intact.

Today most authors interested in craniopharyngioma surgery would in-

Institute of Neurosurgery, University of Milan, Italy
* Ospedale Maggiore, Policlinico, IRCCS, Via F. Sforza 35, Milan, Italy
  Ospedale San Raffaele, Via Olgettina 60, Milan, Italy

deed agree with the view that complete tumor removal is possible and should be the primary goal of any new surgical approach (Fisher et al. 1985; Hoffman et al. 1992; Kahn et al. 1973; Symon and Sprich 1985; Yasargil et al. 1990), although in some instances close relation with hypothalamic tissue may limit radical resection and subtotal surgery would be considered safer.

Modern radiological tools, among which magnetic resonance imaging (MRI) has assumed a primary role, have improved preoperative diagnosis and surgical planning thanks to their impressive anatomopathological description of tumor volume, extension, and boundaries (Baskin and Wilson 1986; Pollack et al. 1988; Yasargil et al. 1990). The ease of early noninvasive diagnoses and the reduction of diagnostic delays may also increase the number of small tumors to deal with, with a greater chance of performing radical surgery with only minor functional derangements. In our series, whereas large tumors were observed in 30% of the patients treated in the period 1976-1982, this figure reduced to 16% in the period 1983-1992.

Although in the majority of the cases MRI studies are able to give correct information regarding the histological nature of the neoplastic growth, the persisting possibility of misdiagnoses should be always kept in mind. The differential diagnosis, for instance, with optic pathway gliomas may in some cases be extremely difficult and may lead to surgical mistakes (Youl et al. 1990). In one patient referred by Sweet (1976) and in one personal case even the direct surgical observation of the involved area led to the false impression of an optic glioma and only at perioperative histological examination of a tumor fragment was the true epithelial nature of the neoplasm able to be defined.

Whenever a tumor cannot be removed totally or subtotal surgery has been intentional, the "benign" craniopharyngioma has a definite, although unpredictable, tendency to recur (Baskin and Wilson 1986; Fisher et al. 1985; Hoffman et al. 1992; Kahn et al. 1973; Symon and Sprich 1985; Yasargil et al. 1990).

Rate of regrowth from tumor remnants and time between primary surgery and symptomatic tumor recurrence also seem rather unpredictable (Baskin and Wilson 1986; Fisher et al. 1985; Hoffman et al. 1992; Kahn et al. 1973; Symon and Sprich 1985; Yasargil et al. 1990). Histological characteristics of the tumor and detailed subclassifications have not been reliable in improving this prognostic task (Adamson et al. 1990; Symon and Sprich 1985).

Treatment of tumor recurrences is still open to debate and a firm consensus has not been reached. Whereas with small asymptomatic tumor remnants observed on MRI a "wait and see" attitude seems to be reasonable whenever serial clinical and MRI follow-up protocols can be scheduled, definite regrowth and/or symptomatic recurrences should be treated.

Whereas secondary surgery is warranted according to many surgeons (Baskin and Wilson 1986; Symon and Sprich 1985; Yasargil et al. 1990), one should be aware that it may be a tremendously difficult and hazardous task to resect a tumor which received external, complementary radiotherapy after primary, subtotal surgery. Furthermore, mortality and morbidity after secondary surgery are usually increased (Baskin and Wilson 1986; Kahn et al. 1973; Katz 1975).

Postoperative adjuvant irradiation was recommended already in 1961 by Kramer and associates (Kramer 1976; Kramer et al. 1961, 1968) and its therapeutic potential recently confirmed by Manaka and coworkers (1985), Baskin and Wilson (1986), and others (Fisher et al. 1985; McMurry et al. 1977).

Symptomatic tapping of predominantly cystic regrowths, possibly combined with stereotactic instillation of yttrium-90 in the tumor cavity (Backlund 1973; Backlund et al. 1972) or stereotactic focused high-beam irradiation of solid tumor remnants with multiple spots (Musolino et al. 1985; Pollack et al. 1988) seem promising alternatives.

Tumor shrinking and quiescence of growth can thus be obtained in some patients although definitive cure cannot be affirmed and the patient must have rigorous, prescheduled, follow-up examinations.

The skilled prescription of substitutive drugs to control endocrine and hydroelectrolytic balance failures furthermore enable us nowadays to restore valid functional levels of a possibly deranged endocrine balance which in the past was one of the major causes of postoperative death (Fisher et al. 1985; Hoffman et al. 1992; Symon and Sprich 1985; Yasargil et al. 1990). Adequate steroid, thyroid, and vasopressin supplements may thus maintain endocrine balance and psychic integrity (Cavazzuti et al. 1983; Galatzen et al. 1991; Grant and Lyen 1982; Hoffman et al. 1992; Symon and Sprich 1985). One should be always aware that endocrine imbalance may worsen psychosocial integrity and great care should be therefore given to perform regular endocrinological evaluations. Nevertheless, weight gain and frank obesity often complicate surgery and may be extremely difficult to cure.

Patients and Methods

We reviewed the clinical charts of all patients who were admitted to the Institute of Neurosurgery of the University of Milano for treatment of a craniopharyngioma from 1976 to 1992 and to the Neurosurgical Department of the Ospedale San Raffaele of Milano from 1988 to 1992. All patients, with the exception of the earliest cases studied with plain skull X-rays, polytomography, and angiography were evaluated with sagittal and coronal computed tomographic scans (CTs) and more recently with CT and MRI. Many of them had also preoperative angiographic examinations, although more recently information obtained by MRI was considered sufficient and angiography not performed. Thorough endocrinological, ophthalmological, and neurological preoperative examinations were conducted before surgery.

As our policy considers surgery the first-choice treatment of the neoplasm and an effort towards radical surgery has always been made, most patients were operated on. In individual cases of huge tumor regrowths, some form of palliative treatment was preferred due to the gross deterioration of neurological and endocrinological status and the unacceptable surgical risk.

Surgical Approach

The pterional route (or subfrontopterional-transsylvian) has been our preferred surgical approach; in our opinion it affords the shortest, most direct route to the parasellar region where the neoplasm originates and is closest to brain structures which must be preserved. Furthermore only a small craniotomy is required; there is only limited brain retraction when the sylvian fissure has previously been opened; there is good visualization of the tumor which may be growing beneath the optic nerves and chiasm; and olfactory nerves need not be damaged.

A unilateral, right-sided flap was usually chosen.

The transsphenoidal route has been considered suitable for primary surgery in predominantly intrasellar infradiaphragmatic tumors with enlarged sellae or in tumors with only limited suprasellar extension.

The ease of reaching intrasellar contents, the low morbidity, and lack of mortality together with the familiarity with the approach led us to choose this route in selected cases. We are fully aware that in individual cases of firm attachment of the tumor to the sellar walls, small remnants with a potential of regrowth may be left behind. In these cases, documented regrowth may be treated by secondary surgery via the pterional route. In most of these cases a correct preoperative diagnosis was made, although in some patients transsphenoidal surgery was chosen for a misdiagnosed pituitary adenoma.

The transcorticotransventricular or the transcallosal approach have been chosen as a first surgical step for those rare, purely intraventricular tumors or as secondary two-stage surgery for tumors extending to the third ventricle when attempts at radical removal were not considered safe using the pterional, translaminaterminalis route. When one of these upper routes is needed, we now always prefer the transcallosal route to avoid postoperative porencephalic cysts and/or seizures.

When operating on children, one should be aware that full maturity of the corpus callosum may be delayed until the third decade.

Combined two-step surgical approaches have been performed whenever radical tumor removal was not achieved with a single procedure. In these cases a second, separate operation has always been conducted after complete recovery from the first procedure.

Shunting Procedures. Ventriculoperitoneal shunts have been implanted pre-operatively when patients were admitted in severe neurological condition, mainly due to prolonged intracranial hypertension secondary to severe obstructive hydrocephalus, and postoperatively whenever hydrocephalus complicated primary or secondary surgical procedures.

Radiotherapy. During the considered period (1976-1992) and especially in the earlier cases of this series, conventional external radiotherapy was advised in patients with major tumor remnants after subtotal tumor removal. The usual total dose was 50-55 Gy.

Tumor Dimensions. Neoplasms were classified as small when their maximal diameter on CT and/or MRI scans was less than 2 cm, as medium size from 2 to 4 cm, and as large when over 4 cm.

Operative Results. Surgical and late follow-up results (mean follow-up time 7 years) were evaluated with a simplified scale. Results were classified as *good* when the patient regained full psychosocial integrity (working ability and psychic integrity), unchanged or improved visual function, and unchanged and well-controlled endocrine functions; as *moderate* when reduction of psychosocial performance was observed or when visual and endocrine functions were unchanged or worsened, and as *poor* when both visual and endocrine functions worsened and significant handicaps were observed at follow-up.

Visual function and endocrine axes were also examined separately and classified as improved, unchanged, or worsened. Postoperative diabetes insipidus has been classified as transitory or permanent. *Complications* of surgery have been finally reported.

Results

The clinical charts of 74 patients, 36 males and 38 females, were reviewed. Of them 22 were in the pediatric age range (0-16 years, mean 11 years) and 52 were adults (mean 41 years). These two groups will first be considered separately. Age and sex distribution and tumor locations are shown in Fig. 1.

Children

Primary surgery was attempted in 19 patients (Tables 1, 2). In about 50% the pterional route was chosen, while in 37% of the cases the transsphenoidal route was considered suitable for primary surgery.

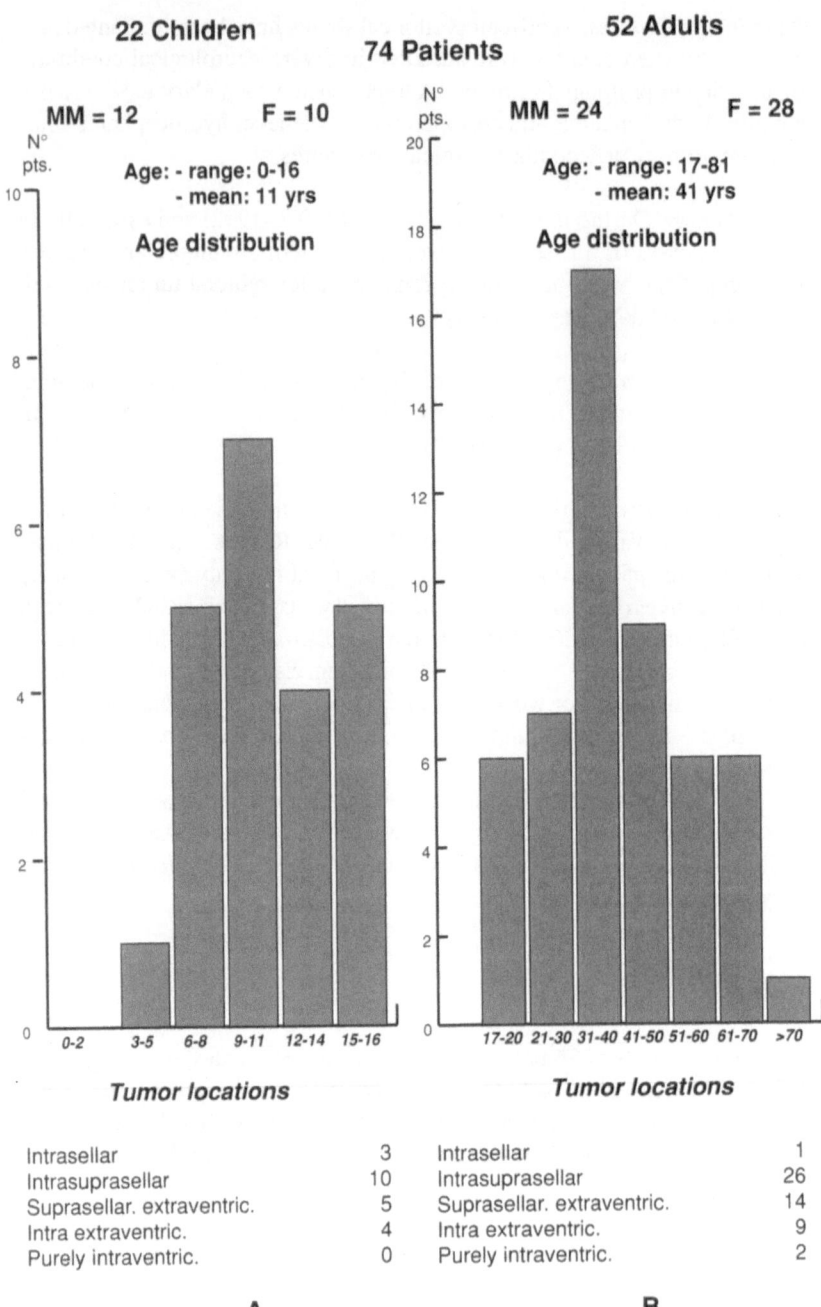

Fig. 1 A, B. General population overview. Age, sex distribution and tumor locations in 74 patients in children (**A**) and adults (**B**)

In three cases of symptomatic tumor recurrence, after a first attempt at radical surgery elsewhere, secondary surgery was conducted via the pterional approach.

Overall, surgery was considered "radical" in 59% of the cases with a direct relation to tumor dimension. Radical removal was indeed achieved in

Table 1. Surgical routes in children

Tumor size	Patients	Secondary surgery	Primary surgery	TNSPH	Pterional	TC/TCTV	Recurrence
Small	7	No	7	6	1	–	No
Medium	8	1	7	1	(1) + 5	1 (TC)	1 Pterional 1 TNSPH
Large	7	2	5	–	(2) + 3	3 [a]	No
Total	22	3	19	7	12	4	

Number of secondary surgeries are indicated in parentheses.
TNSPH, transnasosphenoidal route; TC/TCTV, transcallosal/transcortical-transventricular route
[a] One patient combined TCTV + pterional approach.

Table 2. Surgical results and follow-up in children

Tumor size	Number of cases	Radical removal		Post-operative status	Post-operative management	Recurrence	Secondary surgery	Follow-up
Small < 2 cm	7	Yes	6	G 5, M 1	F.UP 5, RT 1	No	No	G 4, M 2
		No	1	G 1	RT 1	No	No	G 1
Medium 2 - 4 cm	8	Yes	5	G 5	F.UP 5	1	Radical	G 5
		No	3	M 2, G 1	F.UP 2, RT 1	1	Subtotal	G 3
Large > 4 cm	7	Yes	2	D 1, G 1	F.UP 1	No	No	(D 1) G 1
		No	5	G 1, M 3	F.UP 3, RT 2	1	Radical	M 2, P 2
				P 1				D 1
Total	22	Yes	13	D 1, G 14	RT 5	3	3	D 1(D1), G 14
		No	9	M 6, P 1	F.UP 16			M 4, P 2

G, good; M, moderate; P, poor; D, dead; RT, radiotherapy; Pall., palliative therapy (shunt); F.UP, follow-up

86% of the patients harboring small tumors but only in 28.5% of children with large neoplasms.

Good operative results were observed in 64% of the children, moderate in 23%, and poor in 9%. There was one death due to dramatic postoperative hypothalamic failure.

In four of nine patients, in whom tumor removal was not considered radical, treatment was completed with external radiotherapy started shortly after surgery. The remaining five patients with small, asymptomatic remnants were scheduled for clinicoradiological follow-ups. In one patient operated via the transnasosphenoidal route for a misdiagnosed adenoma, external radiotherapy was also performed.

Symptomatic recurrences were all observed within 2 1/2 years from primary surgery and occurred in three children. Three of them were submitted to secondary surgery which was now considered radical in two. Two of the children with symptomatic recurrences were previously submitted to conventional radiotherapy, whereas in one, previous surgery had been considered radical. One of the reoperated children, in whom secondary radical surgery was performed and who needed a postoperative shunt, is now dead due to progressive deterioration of its neurological condition and endocrine failure.

Overall 20 children are still alive, 14 (70%) in good neurological condition, four (20%) moderate, and two (10%) poor. In one of the good survivors an asymptomatic tumor regrowth has been now documented with MRI and type of treatment is under consideration.

Adults

Primary surgery was attempted in 45 patients (Tables 3, 4), mainly (73%) via a pterional approach. In four patients with symptomatic recurrences secondary surgery was performed.

In three patients with recurrence and severe neurological status only palliative treatments were considered possible (two extrathecal shunts and one cystic fluid aspiration after implant of an intracystic catheter connected to an Ommaya reservoir). One of them is now dead due to tumor progression while two survive in poor condition.

Overall, surgery was considered "radical" in 69% of the patients. Whereas radical removal was achieved in all the patients with small tumors it could be performed in only 50% of the patients with large tumors. Operative results were good in 65.6% of the cases, moderate in 19%, and poor in 9.6%.

Operative mortality was 5.8% (cerebral edema and respiratory failure in one, hypothalamic failure in one, and for thrombosis of the basilar artery in a hemophilic patient after factor VIII transfusion).

Table 3. Surgical routes in adults

Tumor size	Patients	Secondary surgery	Primary surgery	TNSPH	Pterional	TC/TCTV	Recurrence
Small	4	No	4	3	1	–	No
Medium	37	4	33	(1) + 5 [b]	(3) + 26	3 (TC)	1 Pterional
							1 Palliative
Large	8	–	8	–	7	1 (TCTV)	No
Total	49 [a]	4	45	9	37	4	

Number of secondary surgeries are indicated in parentheses.
TNSPH, transnasosphenoidal route; TC/TCTV, transcallosal/transcortical-transventricular route
[a] Three patients submitted to palliative treatment.
[b] One patient combined TNSPH + pterional approach.

Table 4. Surgical results and follow-up in adults

Tumor size	Number of cases	Radical removal	Post-operative status	Post-operative management	Recurrence	Secondary surgery	Follow-up
Small < 2 cm	4	Yes 4	G 4	F.UP 4	No	No	G 4
Medium 2 - 4 cm	40	Yes 26	D 2, G 19, M 5	F.UP 24	3	3 [a]	(D 2) G 18, M 5, P 1
		No 11	G 7, M 3, P 1	F.UP 8, RT 3	1	Radical	G 5, M 3, P 1, D 2
		Pall. 3	P 3	RT 2	Persist.	No	P 2, D 1
Large > 4 cm	8	Yes 4	D 1, G 3	F.UP 3	No	No	(D 1)G 3
		No 4	G 1, M 2, P 1	F.UP 2, RT 1, D 1	1	1 [b]	(D 1)M 1 D 2
Total	52	Yes 34	D 3, G 34	RT 6	5	3 [a]	(D 4) D 5[c], G 30
		No 15	M 10, P 5	F.UP 41, D 1		1 [b]	M 9, P 4
		Pall. 3				1 Radical	

G, good; M, moderate; P, poor; D, dead; RT, radiotherapy; Pall., palliative therapy (shunt); F.UP, follow-up
[a] Waiting for decision as to treatment.
[b] Intracystic shunt.
[c] 2 tumor progression, 3 unrelated disease.

Among the patients in whom surgery was considered radical, small, asymptomatic tumor remnants have been detected on follow-up MRI in four. None of them has been treated up to now and all continue to have regular clinico-radiological controls. Palliative treatment was completed with adjuvant radiotherapy in two patients.

Among the 15 patients whose tumor was subtotally removed, four with major tumor remnants were submitted to radiotherapy shortly after surgery. Palliative treatment was completed by adjuvant radiotherapy in two other patients in poor condition.

Notwithstanding radiotherapy one of six patients had a symptomatic recurrence after 2 years. He was submitted to secondary surgery and radical tumor removal was now attained.

In nine patients with small tumor remnants and good surgical outcome a prescheduled clinicoradiological follow-up was organized.

Up to now only one patient had a symptomatic, mainly cystic regrowth, clinically manifested by worsening of previously improved visual function. As this patient is over 60 she was treated with an intracystic shunt and repeated aspiration of cyst contents maintains good visual function.

In three patients an asymptomatic regrowth has now been documented on MRI and decisions on treatment are currently being made. At the last follow-up control (1992) 43 of the 52 observed patients were still alive (three postoperative deaths, two dead due to tumor progression, three dead due to unrelated diseases), 30 are in good condition and fully independent, nine in moderate condition with reduced performance compared to the preoperative status, and four in poor condition. Overall 61% of treated patients maintain a good outcome.

Overview of Results in Both Groups

Transsphenoidal Surgery. Sixteen patients were operated via the transsphenoidal route (seven children and nine adults). In 14 patients primary surgery was considered radical, whereas in two patients secondary surgery using a pterional approach was needed and now afforded radical tumor removal. Notwithstanding surgical judgment in two patients in whom surgery was considered radical, symptomatic regrowth was observed after 2 years. Both have been reoperated via the transphenoidal route and tumor is considered to have been removed completely.

Shunting Procedure. In five patients preoperative shunts and in one case a postoperative shunt was implanted (11.5% of adult patients).

Visual Function and Endocrine Status. See Tables 5 and 6.

Complications. Postoperative complications are reported in Table 7.

Overview of Surgical Results. Considering the whole series of 74 patients observed in the period 1976-1992, complete tumor removal was considered

Table 5. Visual and endocrine function in children and adults

	Children (%)	Adults (%)
Visual function		
• Improved	27	21
• Unchanged	54	68
• Worsened	18	7
Endocrine function		
• Improved	25	20
• Unchanged	65	68
• Worsened	10	12

Table 6. Diabetes insipidus in children and adults

Diabetes insipidus	Children (%)	Adults (%)
Preoperative	27	24
Transitory	39	46
Permanent	36	33

Table 7. Postoperative complications

Complication	Number
Seizures	5
Brain edema	2
Hyphothalamic failure	2
DVT	2
Wound infection	1
Hydrocephalus	1
CSF leak	1
Pulmunary embolism	1
SAH	1
Shock	1
Blindness	1

DVT, deep venous thrombosis; SAH, subarachnoid hemorrhage

as having been achieved in 66% of the 71 operated patients and subtotal tumor removal in 34%, with a postoperative death rate of 5.6%.

Eleven patients (15.5%) were submitted to adjuvant radiotherapy, mainly for major tumor remnants after primary or secondary surgery. Notwithstanding adjuvant irradiation, three of them needed further treatments for symptomatic recurrences. Symptomatic recurrences have been observed and treated in five patients (7%) whereas minor tumor remnants are being followed up in 15 patients (21%). Among them a silent, asymptomatic tendency to tumor regrowth has been observed in four patients and decisions on treatment are currently being discussed.

Sixty-three patients are still alive (four postoperative deaths, four dead due to tumor progression, three due to unrelated diseases). Of them 44 (69%) are considered as having good outcome.

Discussion

Our series confirms that the pessimistic attitude of Northfield (1957) in the late 1950s is no longer justified and that radical surgery of a craniopharyngioma followed by a good quality of life was obtained in 62% of the patients. This improvement is largely due to the appropriate selection of patients, favored by modern preoperative investigational tools, the improvement of pre- and postoperative medical treatments, and the routine use of microsurgical techniques.

Nevertheless, a significant number of patients still have less than favorable results. In large, long-standing tumors extending to the hypothalamus and third ventricle associated with preoperative signs of hypothalamic failure, attempts at radical surgery may further deteriorate functional levels of the patients, especially when tumor adherences with brain tissue cannot be safely cleaved. In these cases the cost of the anatomopathological cure may not be justified considering the ensuing handicaps. In these patients subtotal removal and the attempt at improving visual function seems a reasonable goal, although they are still burdened with the risk of unpredictable regrowths.

For dealing with minor tumor remnants, the availibility of noninvasive and apparently harmless tools such as MRI and CT for prescheduled follow-up neuroradiological controls has made it possible to monitor the tendency of the tumor to regrow since with these modes of imaging small calcified pieces of tumor can be identified and treatment begun when necessary. This might be important for patients who after a first operation present with excellent clinical condition and significant improvement of preoperative neurological deficits. As a matter of fact tumor remnants may in single patients remain quiescent for many years. However, the unpredictability of a possible regrowth requires extreme vigilance, and rigid follow-up protocols should be available.

Radicality of tumor removal as judged during surgery must always be confirmed by MRI and CT studies. In our series we also observed symptomatic tumor recurrences in patients in whom the tumor was considered to have been totally removed. Tumor regrowth may arise from epithelial remnants buried in the sellar walls which were shadowed during the surgical exposure, from calcified and apparently inactive portions left on optic pathways or major vessels, or from residual cells in close relation with a preserved pituitary stalk or hypothalamic tissue.

To avoid overlooking intrasellar portions of the tumor lying beneath and anterior to the chiasm, even after mirror views, we felt in individual cases that it was useful to drill the planum sphenoidale down to the sphenoid, leaving the sphenoidal mucosa intact. The possibility of leaving tumor remnants behind also seems to be increased in mainly cystic tumors in which the thin and friable cyst wall may be torn off and small bits of tumor not completely removed.

In some patients in whom the anatomical integrity of the pituitary stalk could be maintained, the latter may be a potential source of tumor recurrence. Therefore some surgeons feel it is probably better to always excise it. We prefer, however, to leave it intact in the rare cases in which it can be clearly identified and easily separated from the tumor. Serial neuroradiological controls should be therefore particularly strict for these patients.

In any case we suggest that a patient should only be considered cured when complete surgical removal of tumor has been confirmed by at least two postoperative MRI and/or CT controls since tumor regrowths can be observed even after removals which were considered complete at surgery.

With large tumor remnants after surgery during which radical tumor removal was judged as impossible and/or unsafe some form of complementary treatment has to be considered. In our series, covering two decades, conventional external radiotherapy was usually suggested. This choice was justified by the favorable reports of Fisher et al. (1985) and Manaka et al. (1985), and the personal experience of our radiotherapists. Results have been conflicting nevertheless. Whereas tumor shrinking and quiescence has been observed in 73% of the irradiated patients, in 27% of the cases symptomatic tumor recurrences were observed even after full-dose irradiation.

Nowadays, a larger variety of alternative treatments, reported elsewhere in this book, is available and should be considered whenever secondary surgery cannot be performed.

Conclusion

In conclusion we still consider radical tumor removal with the most accurate treatment of endocrine derangements and adequate counseling of patients and their relatives about postoperative problems (among them the avoidance of a natural trend towards obesity) and the best treatment for craniopharyngiomas. Furthermore, surgical results must be confirmed by at least two MRI and/or CT follow-up controls. Whenever radical surgery has been deemed impossible, the availability of alternative treatments nowadays may afford a prolonged symptomatic control of tumor regrowths.

References

Adamson TE, Wiestler OD, Kleihues P, et al (1990) Correlation of clinical and pathological features in surgically treated craniopharyngiomas. J Neurosurg 73:12-17

Backlund EO (1973) Studies on craniopharyngiomas. III. Stereotaxic treatment with intracystic yttrium-90. Acta Chir Scand 139:237-247

Backlund EO, Johansson L, Sorby B (1972) Studies on craniopharyngiomas. II. Treatment by stereotaxis and radiosurgery. Acta Chir Scand 138:749-759

Baskin DS, Wilson CB (1986). Surgical management of craniopharyngiomas. J Neurosurg 65:22-27

Cavazzuti V, Fisher EG, Welch K, et al (1983) Neurological and psychophysiological sequelae following different treatment of craniopharyngiomas in children. J Neurosurg 59:409-417

Cushing HW (1932) Intracranial tumors. Notes upon a series of two thousand verified cases with surgical mortality percentages pertaining theretho. Thomas, Springfield, p 97

Fisher EG, Welch K, Belli JA, et al (1985) Treatment of craniopharyngiomas in children: 1972-1981. J Neurosurg 62:496-501

Galatzen A, Nofar E, Halachm BN, et al (1981) Intellectual and psychosocial functions of children, adolescents and young adults before and after operation for craniopharyngiomas. Child Care Health Dev 7:307-316

Grant DB, Lyen K (1982) Hypopitituarism after surgery for craniopharyngioma. Child Brain 9:201-204

Hoffman HJ, Hendrick EB, Humphreys RP, et al (1977) Management of craniopharyngiomas in children. J Neurosurg 47:218-227

Hoffman HJ, De Silva M, Humphreys RP (1992) Aggressive surgical management of craniopharyngiomas in children. J Neurosurg 76:47-52

Kahn EA, Gosh HH, Seeger JF, et al (1973) Forty-five years experience with craniopharyngiomas. Surg Neurol 1:5-12

Katz EL (1975) Late results of radical excision of craniopharyngiomas in children. J Neurosurg 42:86-90

Kramer S (1976) Craniopharyngiomas: the best treatment is conservative surgery and postoperative radiation therapy. In: Marley TP (ed) Current controversies in neurosurgery. Saunders, Philadelphia, pp 336-343

Kramer S, McKissock W, Coucannon JP (1961) Craniopharyngiomas. Treatment by combined surgery and radiation therapy. J Neurosurg 18:217-226

Kramer S, Southard H, Hansfield C (1968) Radiotherapy in the management of craniopharyngiomas: further experiences and late results. Am J Roentgenol Radium Ther Nucl Med 103:44-52

Lapras C, Palet JD, Mattolise C, et al (1987) Craniopharyngiomas in childhood. Analysis of 42 cases. Progr Exp Tumor Res 30:350-358

Manaka S, Teramoto A, Takakura K (1985) The efficacy of radiotherapy for craniopharyngiomas. J Neurosurg 62:648-656

Matson DD (ed) (1969) Neurosurgery of infancy and childhood, 2nd edn. Thomas, Springfield

Matson D.D, Cligler JF Jr (1969) Management of craniopharyngiomas in childhood. J Neurosurg 27:52-79

McMurry FG, Hardy RW, Donh DF, et al (1977) Longterm results in the management of craniopharyngiomas. Neurosurgery 1:238-241

Musolino A, Munari C, Blond S, et al (1985) Traitement stereotaxique des cystes expansifs de craniopharyngiomes pour irradiation endocavitaire Beta (Re 186; Au 198; Y 90). Neurochirurgie 31:69-178

Northfield DWC (1957) Rathke-pouch tumors. Brain 80:293-312

Pollack IF, Lunsford LD, Slamovits TL (1988) Stereotaxic intracavitary irradiation for cystic craniopharyngiomas. J Neurosurg 68:227-233

Sweet WH (1976) Radical surgical treatment of craniopharyngiomas. Clin Neurosurg 27:52-79

Symon L, Sprich W (1985) Radical excision of craniopharyngiomas: results in 20 patients. J Neurosurg 62:174-181

Yasargil MG, Curcic M, Kis M, et al (1990) Total removal of craniopharyngiomas. Approaches and long term results in 144 patients. J Neurosurg 73:3-11

Youl BD, Plant GT, Steven JH, et al (1990) Three cases of craniopharyngiomas showing optic tract hypersignal on MRI. Neurology 40:1416-1419

Some Problems of Craniopharyngioma Treatment

A. N. Konovalov

Over the past decades the results of surgical treatment of craniopharyngiomas have substantionally improved due to precise diagnosis using computed tomography (CT) and magnetic resonance imaging (MRI), better surgical technique, and more effective postoperative intensive care. Some neurosurgeons have achieved very impressive and promising results (Suzuki et al.1984; Symon and Sprich 1985; Yasargil et al. 1987; Choux et al.1991). In spite of this, the treatment of craniopharyngiomas as a whole still presents one of the most serious neurosurgical problems.

At the Moscow Burdenko Neurosurgical Institute, to which patients with the most difficult cerebral tumors are admitted from all over the country, I have operated on about 700 patients with craniopharyngiomas. This experience has convinced me that surgery cannot solve all the problems of patients bearing these dangerous tumors. The safe and radical removal of some tumor still presents serious problems, the number of complications is still high, and the recurrence rate is also quite remarkable after attempted radical tumor resection. Taking this consideration into account I will address in this paper the problems which are still far from being finally solved.

The first problem is the *classification of craniopharyngiomas*. There are different groups of craniopharyngiomas and the results of treatment in these groups vary greatly. A generally accepted division of craniopharyngiomas into prechiasmal and retrochiasmal is, in our opinion, not very appropriate as it does not define the tumor third ventricle relationship.

In the Burdenko Institute we differentiate three main groups of craniopharyngiomas: endosuprasellar, suprasellar-extraventricular (some of them are in a retrochiasmal location), and craniopharayngiomas penetrating into the third ventricle. A separation of the group of the third ventricle craniopharyngiomas seems to us very important as approaches to this tumor are the most difficult and quite often they can be removed only when different approaches are combined. In this group of craniopharyngiomas results are worse than those gained in tumors which do not penetrate the third ventricle.

Burdenko Institute, Fadeev Street 5, Moscow 125047

Endosuprasellar Craniopharyngiomas

Tumors in endosuprasellar locations are the most favorable for successful removal. Some of them can be effectively removed via the transsphenoidal route both in adults and in children. In the past decade 40 endosellar and endosuprasellar craniopharyngiomas were removed at the Burdenko Neurosurgical Institute using this approach (constituting about 3% of all transsphenoidal tumor removals).

Still, the transcranial (subfrontal or pterional) approach in the surgery of these tumors is the most common. For endosellar craniopharyngiomas with a large extrasellar expansion we try, if possible, to preserve the pituitary stalk and the vascular connection with the remnants of the pituitary. To achieve this the suprasellar capsule of the tumor is divided into two layers: external, which is a distended diaphragm of the sella, and internal, a proper capsule of craniopharyngiomas. After the radical extirpation of the endo- and suprasellar part of the tumor, we suture the external layer of the capsule above the sella to reconstruct the normal anatomic relations and prevent the dislocation of the chiasma and hypothalamus in the sellar cavity, which can be very large.

Third Ventricle Craniopharyngiomas

In some cases the tumor is located mainly in the cavity of the third ventricle; in others the tumor occupies the third ventricle and spreads outside of it. Modern techniques, primarily magnetic resonance imaging (MRI), permit differentiation of these groups of tumors. There are different ways of approaching tumors located in the third ventricle: via the lamina terminalis, through the corpus callosum, by interhemispheric and pterional routes.

In Table 1 those approaches to the third ventricle craniopharyngiomas are presented which I have employed. One can see that they are mainly reached through the corpus callosum or via a subfrontal route when the tumor is removed through the lamina, terminalis or opticocarotid triangle. The pterional approach to which we resort more often now does not seriously differ from the subfrontal approach. In Table 1 one can also see that the combined approaches are quite commonly used: subfrontal or pterional in combination with transcallosal.

We usually start with the transcallosal approach: if the tumor cannot be completely removed by this route the basal extraventricular part of craniopharyngioma can be reached with the help of subfrontal or pterional craniotomy (Figs. 1, 2).

The corpus callosum is divided between the pericallosal arteries with a midline incision of 1-1.5 cm in length. After that the tumor may be removed

Table 1. Surgical approaches to craniopharyngiomas of the third ventricle

Approaches	Children (n)	Adults (n)	Total (n)
Transcallosal	88	33	121
• combined	- 25	- 3	- 28
Transcortical	5	8	13
• combined	- 4	- 7	- 11
Subfrontal and pterional	65	31	96
Subtemporal	9	5	14
• combined	- 1	- 1	- 2
Total	167	77	244

through one or both foramina of Monro, which usually are enlarged by the tumor. To use both foramina it is necessary to make a window in the septum pellucidum. The tumor can also be rached via the roof of the third ventricle by dividing the columna fornicis. This approach is preferable when there is a third ventricle cavity (which can be revealed on CT and MRI scans) or when the tumor bulging in the upper compartment of the ventricle distends the fornix, which makes it very simple to split the column. In our experience there are quite often tight adherences between the tumor capsule and walls of the third ventricle, especially laterally and anteriorly. In some cases the tumor adheres to the edges of the foramina of Monro and to the root of the third ventricle.

The posterior walls of the ventricle in the region of the aqueduct are usually free from adherences with the tumor capsule. We start by evacuating the cystic content and removing its solid part. More difficult is the removal of the basal suprasellar part of the tumor, which is usually calcified and may be very strong, but without that it is impossible to achieve radical tumor resection.

In our experience, the transcallosal approach (including the combined approaches) permits a more radical tumor removal than do the subfrontal or pterional approaches, when the tumor is reached through the lamina terminalis and the opticocarotid triangle.

I would like to emphasize that there is no ideal method of surgical management of third ventricle craniopharyngiomas. A surgeon has to vary approaches, combine them, and try new ones. In spite of a good deal of experience with the transcallosal approach, which may provide favorable conditions for radical tumor removal, I do not consider it an option for surgery of third ventricle craniopharyngiomas and, in agreement with Samii (from a report on skull base surgery during the Skull-Base Congress in Hannover, Germany, 1992 and from personal communication), recommend removing them

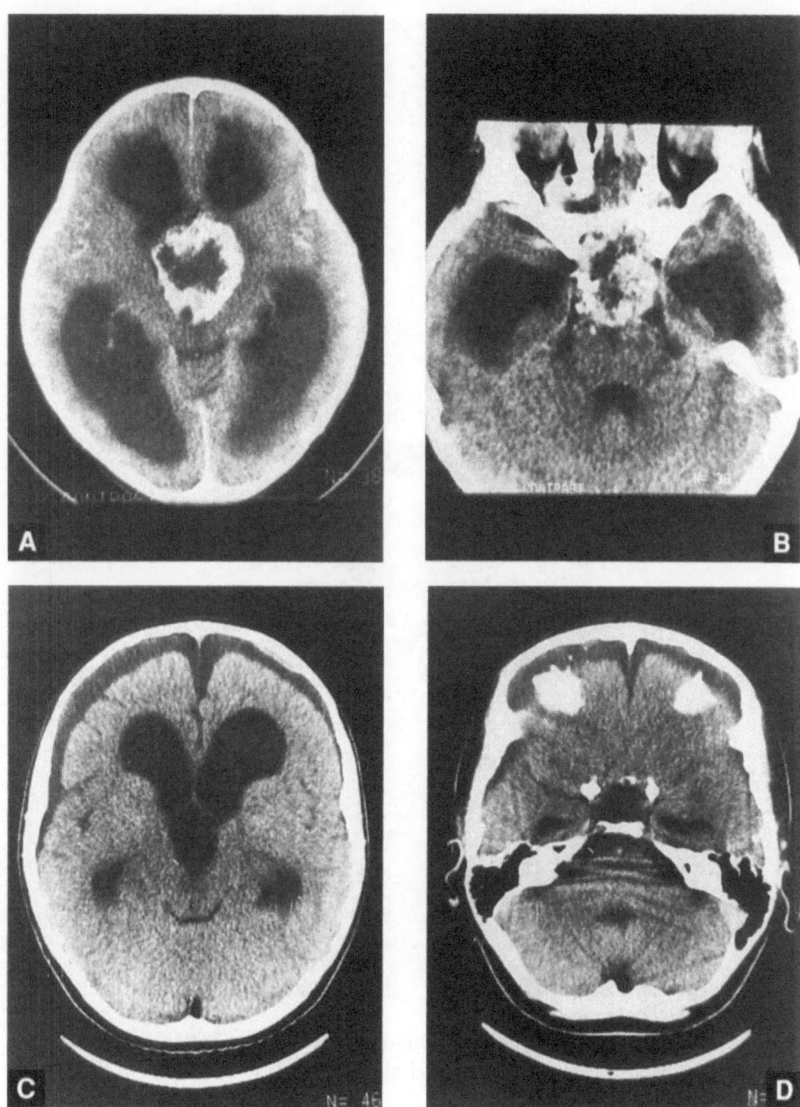

Fig. 1 A-D. Third ventricle craniopharyngioma before *(A, B)* and after *(C, D)* trans-callosal removal

using a bifrontal basal approach with resection of the orbital rim and the base of the nose. Beside the selection of an appropriate approach, management of third ventricle craniopharyngiomas presents some additional problems.

Hydrocephalus is one of the most common accompanying conditions in craniopharyngiomas extending into the third ventricle; it is a sequela of oc-

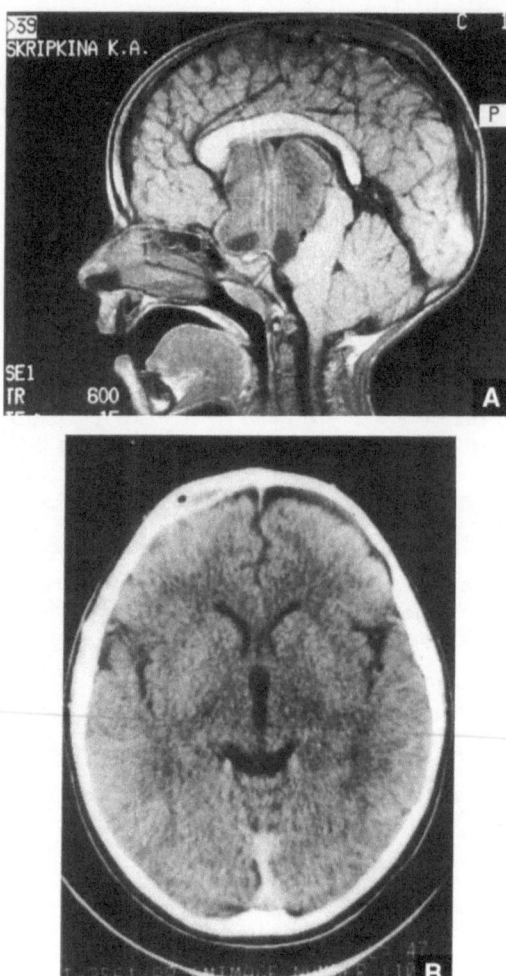

Fig. 2 A, B. Third ventricle craniopharyngioma before (**A**) and after removal with the he]p of combined-transcallosal-pterional-approach (**B**)

clusion in the foramina of Monro or aqueduct (or both). Hydrocephalus facilitates access to the tumor but at the same time it may cause serious complications after the tumor is removed: brain collapse or subdural air, CSF fluid,
and blood collections. In some cases an additional surgical procedure such
as subdural hematoma drainage becomes necessary. This is why it is better
to start the treatment with shunting when the ventricles are too large. But
after that it is necessary to check changes in the ventricular volume and to
operate on the patient before the ventricles become small or even collapse.

We have also found that in some cases cystic craniopharyngiomas begin to enlarge rapidly after shunting the ventricles, probably due to changes in intracranial volume-pressure relations.

Another serious problem is possible damage to the hypothalamus, especially when the tumor is solid, calcified, and firmly adhered to the floor and the walls of the third ventricle. In such cases, the transcallosal approach has some advantages as the tumor is moved under direct visual control. Possible preservation of the vascularization of the hypothalamus is of great importance, the problem being that the tumor and the hypothalamus have the same sources of vascularization. Our experience has shown that it is relatively easier to preserve these vessels by removing the tumor via the transcallosal approach. When any of these vessels are damaged, it is better not to coagulate them and to stop the bleeding with gelfoam.

The next matter of great importance is change in the brain circulation, which occurs quite often after removing craniopharyngiomas in general and especially when craniopharyngiomas are located in the third ventricle.

We have found that sometimes after the successful radical removal of the tumor, the patient's condition is quite satisfactory. He or she is alert, without any serious signs of hypothalamic lesion except for diabetis insipidus, which is the most common postoperative complication. But after several days the patient becomes drowsy and somnolent and signs of brain damage such as convulsions, pyramidal pareses, speech disturbances, and so on become evident. At the same time serious changes in the water-electrolyte balance are evident. In the most severe cases patients die. Postmortem examination performed by A.G. Korshunov have revealed the spread and severe changes in the brain circulation: thrombosis of small and large arteries and veins, dissecting aneurysms, decomposition of the elastic membrane etc. Ischemic lesions in various regions of the brain are the result of these disturbances in cerebral vascularization.

Similar but less pronounced vascular lesions were revealed in patients with craniopharyngiomas who died without surgery. It is difficult to give an exact explanation of this phenomenon caused by the damage to the hypothalamus (chronic and acute). It might be that the pathological secretion of vasoactive peptides in combination with water-electrolyte imbalance forms the basis for cerebral circulation disturbances, as mentioned above.

The next serious problem is the *management of giant* (mostly cystic) *craniopharyngiomas*. Giant craniopharyngiomas constitute about 20% of all pediatric craniopharyngiomas treated in the Burdenko Neurosurgical Institute. They can belong to any group of craniopharyngiomas, but most often to those which develop at the level of the pituitary stalk and lie above the sella but beneath the base of the brain. They can form giant cysts in the anterior, middle, and posterior fossa (Fig. 3) and penetrate deeply into the brain, into the lateral and the third ventricles. It may be one cyst or several separated cysts with different contents.

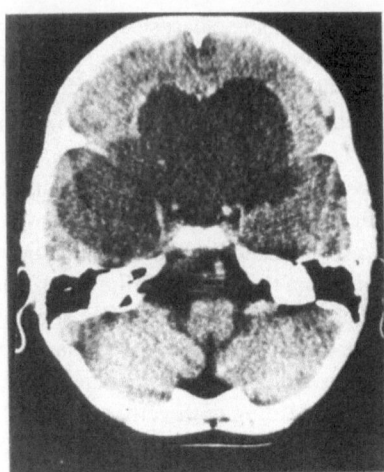

Fig. 3. Giant cystic craniopharyngioma

It must be particularly emphasized that clinical manifestation of some giant cystic craniopharyngiomas in children may seriously differ from the main group of craniopharyngiomas-signs of hypothalamic damage which are so typical for craniopharyngiomas may be absent. The postmortem examination in some of these cases has revealed that the pituitary stalk and hypothalamus are not damaged but only displaced by the tumor which spreads into the subarachnoid space.

The capsule of these tumors may be strong and well developed, which facilitates tumor removal, or it can be very thin, transparent, and consist practically of the basal membrane and a single layer of epithelial cells. The capsule of such craniopharyngiomas envelops the chiasma, optic and other cranial nerves, and the main basal arteries and their branches like a muff, which makes their radical removal extremely difficult. Even when a small amount of the tumor capsule is left unremoved, it may become a source for giant cyst recurrence.

We have investigated other modes of giant craniopharyngioma treatment. In five cases of instillation of yttrium oleate in the cysts positive results were achieved in four; a follow-up from 6 months to 3 years revealed that cysts became smaller, but at the same time the degree of the calcification of their walls increased. Irradiation of recurrent cyst after surgical removal may result in a stabilization of the process.

We also have some experience with the instillation of bleomycin through the Ommaya system. Eleven patients with 16 cysts were treated with this technique: improvement or stabilization of cyst progression was only achieved in six patients. In other patients we have observed different complications: meningism, seizures, deterioration of vision, leak of bleomycin along the catheter in the ventricular system or into the subarachnoid space, and rapid reaccumulation of cysts.

Repeated punctures of large cysts or their drainage with the help of the Ommaya system may only help temporarily. We drain cysts before direct surgery to improve a patient's condition and diminish the size of the cysts. In general, all the above-mentioned methods may result in temporary improvement or stabilization of the process. Only the radical removal of these tumors (although difficult and rather dangerous) may cure or provide long-lasting improvement of the patient's condition.

Surgical approaches to giant cystic craniopharyngiomas vary, depending on the precise localization of the tumor. In our practice we use frontal (uni- and bilateral), pterional, subtemporal-transtentorial, occipital paramedian, transcallosal ventricular-transcortical approaches, and combinations of them. In every case hours of meticulous microsurgical dissection are necessary to separate the tumor from vessels, cranial nerves, and important brain structure and to achieve radical removal.

Beside the localization and the size of the tumor results of craniopharyngioma treatment depend on the stage of the illness and the effectiveness of previous correction of endocrine dysfunction.

At the Burdenko Neurosurgical Institute we quite often have had to operate on patients in a final phase of the illness- blind and exhausted, with pronounced signs of endocrine insufficiency. Many of them were previously, unsuccessfully treated. Results in these cases are worse than in patients operated on during the early stages of the illness with previous adequate medical correction.

Our experience shows that patients in whom radical surgery is the most risky are aged patients, especially with tumors of the third ventricle, and patients with recurrent craniopharyngiomas. Further improvement of neurosurgical technique, better understanding of the causes of the main complications, and outlining the surgical groups at greatest risk are necessary to achieve better results in craniopharyngioma treatment.

References

Choux M, Lena G, Genitori L (1991) Le craniopharyngiome de l'enfant. Neurochirurgie 37 [Suppl 1]:1-174

Konovalov AN (1994) Surgery of cranioharyngiomas and gliomas of the chiasma and the third ventricle. In: Samii M (ed) Skull base surgery. First Int Skull Base Congr, Hannover 1992. Karger, Basel, pp 408-411

Suzuki J, Katakura R, Mori T (1984) Interhemispheric approach through the lamina terminalis to the tumor of the anterior part of the III ventricle. Surg Neurol 22:157-163

Symon L, Sprich W (1985) Radical excision of craniopharyngiomas. Results of 20 patients. J Neurosurg 62:174-151

Yasargil MG, Reody PJ, Roth P (1987) Combined approaches. In: Apuzzo MLJ (ed) Surgery of the third ventricle. Williams and Wilkins, Baltimore

Role of the Transsphenoidal Approach in the Surgical Treatment of Craniopharyngiomas

G. Nicola, G. Lasio, L. Valentini, S. Visintini, and C. L. Solero

Introduction

During the first 10 years of this century the transsphenoidal (TNS) approach was developed to treat pituitary tumors (Cushin 1932), but the limitations of this route in removing tumors other than pituitary adenomas were soon recognized. Craniopharyngiomas are rarely confined to the sella turcica (Carmel 1985); their capsule is frequently firmly adherent to suprasellar vascular and nervous structures and their consistency is variable, but often quite hard. Today, the preferred treatment of craniopharyngiomas is radical surgical removal at the first attempt (Yasargil et al. 1990; Hoffman et al. 1992), and given these premises the question arises as to whether the TNS approach has a role in the treatment of these tumors.

Material and Methods

From 1972 to 1992, 92 patients were operated on by the senior author (G.N.) for craniopharyngioma. To analyze the series we have adopted the classification proposed by Yasargil et al. in 1990. Tumors were classified as: type A, purely intrasellar-infradiaphragmatic; type B, intra- and suprasellar, infra- and supradiaphragmatic; type C, supradiaphragmatic, parachiasmatic, extraventricular; type D, intra- and extraventricular; type E, paraventricular; and type F, purely intraventricular. In rare cases craniopharyngiomas can be located epidurally (sphenoid sinus and clivus or middle fossa) and even extracranially.

In our series 42 tumors were classified as type B, 25 as type C, and 13 as type D. Only 12 tumors belonged in the other categories, and only three tumors were type A craniopharyngiomas (3.3%).

The TNS approach was used in 12 cases (11%). Three tumors were classified as type A; in two other cases the TNS approach was used to remove a

Div. of Neurosurgery, Istituto Nazionale Neurologico "C. Besta", Via Celoria 11, 20133 Milan, Italy

sphenoidal extension of the craniopharyngioma, whose intracranial component had been resected previously (Figs. 1-3). In three cases the TNS ap-

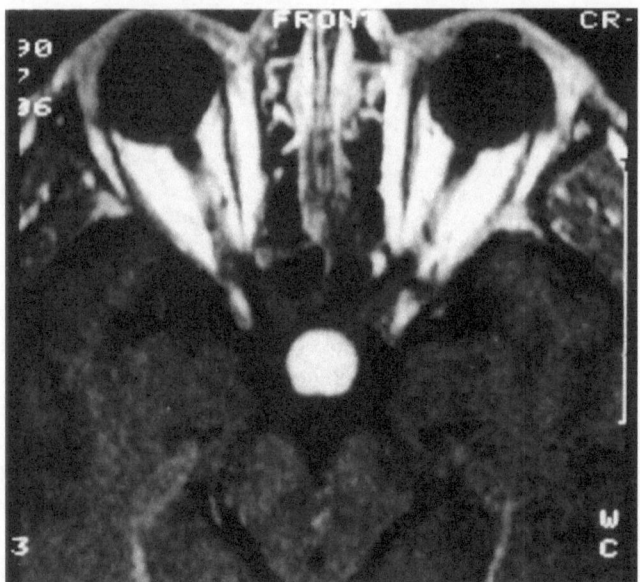

Fig. 1. CT scan of type A craniopharyngioma

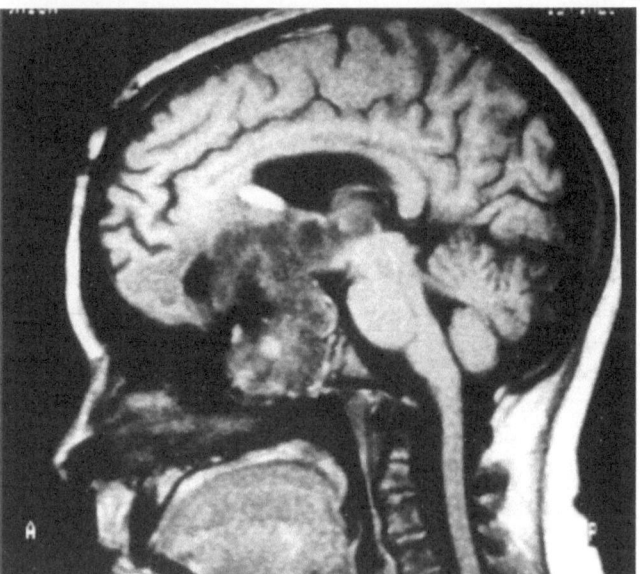

Fig. 2. Preoperative T1-weighted sagittal MRI section, showing intra-extra-cranial,
huge recurrent craniopharyngioma

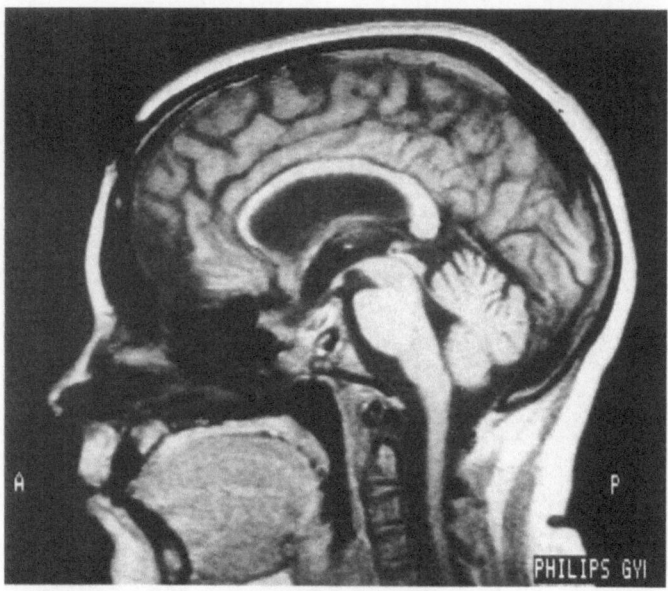

Fig. 3. Postoperative T1-weighted MRI scan after transcranial and transsphenoidal operations

proach was used to palliate symptoms of endosuprasellar, mainly cystic tumors, in patients requiring emergency decompression of the optic pathways, or in patients in poor general condition or who refused craniotomy. These patients were then treated with conventional radiotherapy. In four cases the TNS approach was chosen because of an incorrect radiological diagnosis of pituitary adenoma (Figs. 4, 5). There was no mortality and no endocrinological or neurological morbidity. Total removal of the lesion was achieved in seven cases. Recurrence appeared in three of them (43%), with a minimum follow-up of 2 years.

Recurrences occurred in one type A craniopharyngioma and in two patients with misdiagnosis. No recurrence has been detected, up to now, in the two patients who had both transcranial and TNS operations; they were not considered in the group of "total removal" surgery anyway.

Discussion and Conclusions

The strategy of the senior author in the treatment of craniopharyngiomas is to attempt total removal of the tumor at first surgery rather than to risk repeated operations or to prescribe postoperative radiation therapy with its attending side effects. From our series it appears that total removal of the

tumor was reached in seven cases out of 12 so operated on (58%). These
results compare favorably with previously reported series (Hardy and

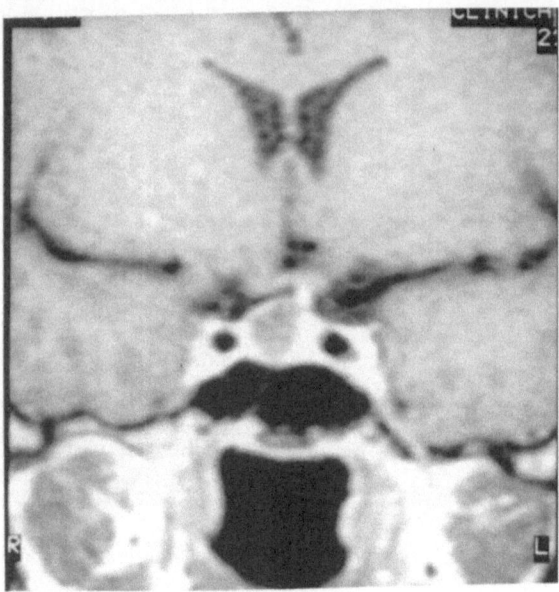

Fig. 4. Preoperative MRI scan of type A craniopharyngioma (neuroradiological diagnosis of pituitary adenoma)

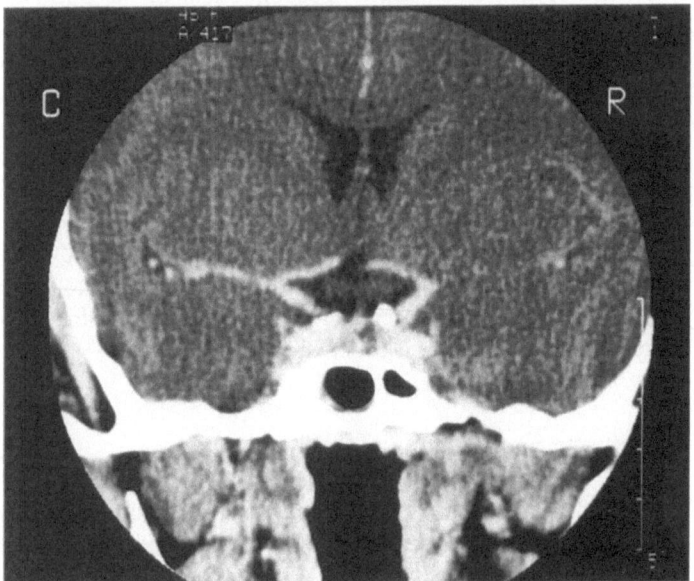

Fig. 5. Postoperative CT scan of patient seen in Fig. 4

Vezina 1976; Konig et al. 1986; Laws 1980; Tanaka and Kobayashi 1989), and in any series we have analyzed the percentage of craniopharyngiomas approached transsphenoidally varies from 4% to 30% (Baskin and Wilson 1986; Tomita 1988; Yasargil et al. 1990; Choux et al. 1991). The percentage of recurrences, in our series, however, is unacceptably high (43%).

The TNS approach has advantages and disadvantages: this approach permits a fast decompression of the optic pathways and the improvement of visual function is better and more complete (Grisoli et al. 1982; Konig et al. 1986; Laws 1980). Moreover, the endocrinological functions are better preserved after surgery. Konig showed visual improvement in 94% of the patients operated on via the TSN route, compared to 65% obtained in the patients operated on transcranially.

The main disadvantage of the approach rests on the difficulty of completely removing the tumor, in particular when the lesion extends outside the limits of the sella turcica, is firmly adherent to suprasellar vascular and nervous structures, or is of a hard consistency. In these situations the surgeon, working through a deep, confined surgical field, has to pull the tumor: this maneuver is very hazardous without any direct visual control. The approach is rendered even more difficult when the sella is not enlarged and in children, in whom the sphenoidal sinus is not pneumatized. A high speed drill can be helpful in this situation.

In conclusion, we think that the TNS approach is indicated only for intrasellar craniopharyngiomas (3% of our series, 15% of the Choux review). It

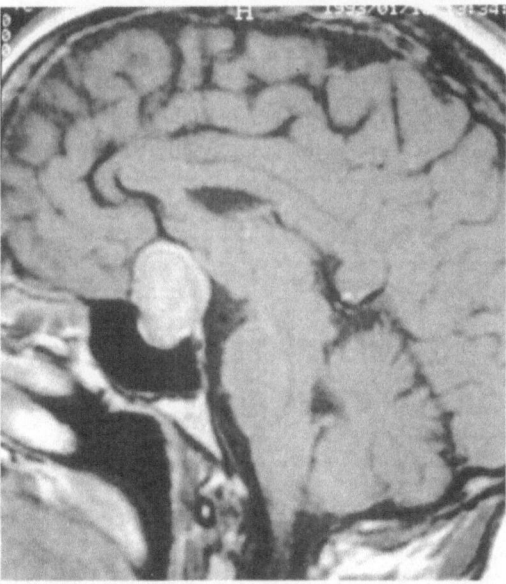

Fig. 6. Preoperative Tl-weighted MRI scan of a presumed pituitary adenoma

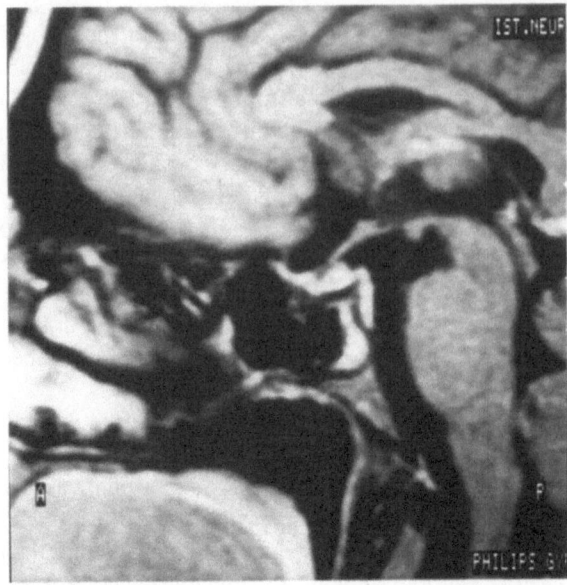

Fig. 7. Postoperative MRI control: complete removal. Histological diagnosis: craniopharyngioma

can be useful when an emergency decompression of the optic pathways is needed and the tumor has a large median suprasellar cystic component. In some cases it can precede or follow a transcranial approach to remove a basal extension of the tumor, particularly in the sphenoid sinus, as in two of our cases.

Sometimes the use of this approach has been completely successful even when not indicated, but this is just a lucky and fortuitous occurrence (Figs. 6, 7).

References

Baskin DS, Wilson CB (1986) Surgical management of craniopharyngiomas. J Neurosurg 65:22-27

Carmel PW (1985) Craniopharyngiomas. In: Wilkins RH, Rengachary SS (eds) Neurosurgery. Mc Graw-Hill, New-York, p 905

Choux M, Lena G, Genitori L (1991) Le craniopharyngiome de l'enfant. Neurochir, 37:[Suppl 1]

Cushing H (1932) Pituitary body, hypothalamus and parasympathetic nervous system. Thomas, Springfield

Grisoli F, Vincentelli F, Farnarier P et al (1982) Transsphenoidal microsurgery in the management of non-pituitary tumors of the sella turcica. In: Brock M (ed) Modern neurosurgery, vol 1. Springer, Berlin Heidelberg New York, pp193-204

Hardy J, Vezina JL (1976) Transsphenoidal surgery of intracranial neoplasms. Adv Neurol 15:261-274

Hoffman HJ, De Silva M, Humphreys RP, et al (1992) Aggressive surgical management of craniopharyngiomas in children. J Neurosurg 76:47-52

Konig A, Ludecke DK, Herrmann HD (1986) Transnasal surgery in the treatment of craniopharyngiomas. Acta Neurochir 83:1-7

Laws ER Jr (1980) Transsphenoidal microsurgery in the management of craniopharyngioma. J Neurosurg 52:661-666

Tanaka T, Kobayashi T (1989) The results of treatment of craniopharyngioma in 33 children. No Shinkei Geka 16:845-850

Tomita T (1988) Management of craniopharyngiomas in children. Pediatr Neurosci 14:204-211

Yasargil MG, Curcic M, Kis M, et al (1990) Total removal of craniopharyngiomas. Approaches and long-term results in 144 patients. J Neurosurg 73:3-11

Surgical Treatment of Craniopharyngiomas

G. Cantore, V. Esposito, and B. Fraioli

Introduction

Treatment of craniopharyngiomas is still controversial, in spite of the unceasing improvements in neuroradiological diagnosis, neuroanesthesia, surgical technique, and pharmacological therapy. The complete surgical removal of the tumor is undoubtedly the gold standard (Guidetti and Fraioli 1979; Hoffman et al. 1977; Katz 1975; Lapras et al. 1987; Shapiro et al. 1979; Sweet 1976; Symon and Sprich 1985; Yasargil et al. 1990); however, sometimes this is an impossible goal to achieve, because of unacceptably high surgical risks. On the other hand, subtotal removal is associated with a remarkable incidence of recurrences; several authors advocate postoperative radiotherapy for these cases (Baskin and Wilson 1986; Carmel et al. 1982; Fisher et al. 1985; Guidetti and Fraioli 1979; Manaka et al: 1985; Richmond et al. 1980; Shapiro et al. 1979; Viramuthu and Benton 1983), but others argue against it because of "its unpredictable side effects" (Yasargil et al. 1990). Brachytherapy (Mundinger and Hoefer 1974), stereotactic radiosurgery (Backlund et al. 1972; Backlund 1973b; Colombo et al. 1985; Leksell 1983; Valentino 1988), intracavitary radiotherapy (Backlund 1973a, 1988; Bond et al. 1965; Julow et al. 1985; Kobayashi et al. 1981; Leksell et al. 1967; Munari et al. 1988; Pollack et al. 1988; Strauss et al. 1982) and chemotherapy (Broggi et al. 1988; Takahashi et al. 1985), and drainage of craniopharyngioma cysts (Spaziante et al. 1989) have all been considered as an alternative or additional treatment to open surgery. Good results were reported for each of these alternative procedures, but only a small number of patients treated are available for long-term analysis. At present, the real value of these techniques and their late adverse effects remain to be assessed (Pang 1993). Therefore, our first-choice treatment is open surgery. Our series includes patients treated via several surgical approaches: frontotemporal or pterional, subfrontal uni-or bilateral, subtemporal, transcallosal, transphenoidal, transmaxillosphenoidal, stereotactic. A small group of pa-

Dept. of Neurological Sciences, University "La Sapienza", Div. Neurosurgery, Viale dell'Università 30/A, 00185 Rome, Italy

tients needed combined approaches, most of them for removal of giant tumors; in selected cases, we found it useful to combine a frontotemporal approach with a basal bifrontal one. The majority of our patients were operated on via a frontotemporal approach; in our experience, it allowed a radical and safe removal of the great majority of craniopharyngiomas.

Surgical Technique

In order to achieve a wide exposure of the chiasmatic region we combine subfrontal and pterional approaches, performing a frontotemporal approach from the nondominant side (with the exception of particular cases) extended frontally close to the midline. The frontobasal burr hole is placed just beside the superior sagittal sinus, flush with the anterior cranial fossa floor. After dural incision and exposure of the chiasmatic region, the prechiasmatic and right carotid cisterns are opened widely. Further arachnoid dissection is carried toward the sylvian fissure, which is extensively separated. The frontal lobe is thus freed from its arachnoidal adhesions with the temporal lobe and vascular and optic structures. Hence, only a minimal pressure is required on the frontal lobe retractor to gain a wide exposure of the chiasmatic region. The surgical microscope can be used along an angle measuring about 90° from a plane very close to that in which the falx cerebri lies to a plane perpendicular to the falx itself (Fig. 1). All the main surgical spaces, such as the interoptic, opticocarotid, right laterocarotid and the lamina terminalis, are easily visualized and accessible. The subfrontal angulation of the surgical microscope (that is, along a plane as close as possible to the falx cerebri) allows adequate visualization of the vascular and optic structures contralateral to the side of the approach. Moreover, the lamina terminalis surface can be widely exposed and is easier to distinguish from the optic structures bordering it anteriorly and laterally. In contrast, the pterional angulation of the surgical microscope allows better visualization of the posterior parts of the tumor, even under the optic tracts. Intratumoral debulking of the mass and careful dissection of the tumor capsule from vascular and nervous structures of the suprasellar region have allowed radical removal of the great majority of craniopharyngiomas: in some cases, we prefer to leave only small fragments of tumor capsule in situ, because of their dense adhesions to the hypothalamus or to the vessels of the posterior cerebral circle.

Illustrative Cases

We present two case studies of patients operated on by the technique described.

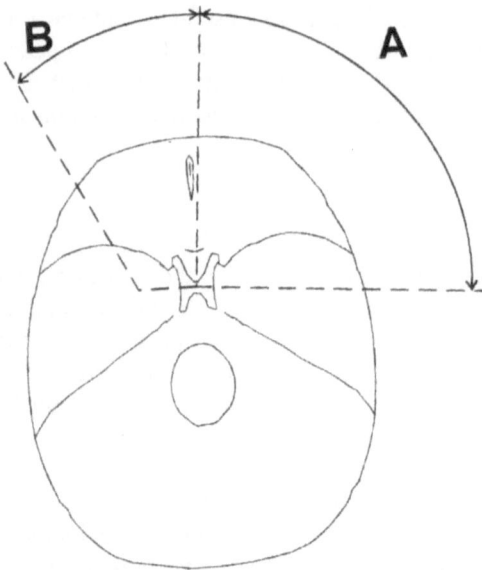

Fig. 1 A, B. (**A**) The surgical angle available with our frontotemporal approach to the chiasmatic region. The surgical microscope can be used along an angle measuring about 90° from a plane very close to that in which the falx cerebri lies to a plane perpendicular to the falx itself. The keys to achieving this exposure are a wide opening of the sylvian fissure and a frontobasal burr hole as close as possible to midline. (**B**) When needed during surgery, the surgical angle can be furtherly widened by performing a controlateral frontal bone flap.

Case 1. A 60-year-old woman presented with a 2-month history of diabetes insipidus and bilateral visual loss. Enhanced cerebral magnetic resonance imaging (MRI) showed a supraretrosellar tumor with solid and cystic components (Fig. 2). A right frontotemporal approach allowed total resection of the tumor. The retrosellar portion was resected through the lamina terminalis. The pituitary stalk was divided because of neoplastic invasion. Postoperative, contrast-enhanced MRI confirmed complete removal of the craniopharyngioma (Fig. 3).

Case 2. A fully sexually developed 12-years-old girl presented with a 4-month history of diabetes insipidus and bilateral visual loss. Cerebral, contrast-enhanced MRI showed a bulky tumor with large supraretrosellar extension (Fig. 4). The left lateral ventricle was markedly enlarged because of obstruction of the foramen of Monro. Enhanced cerebral computed tomography (CT) proved that the tumor was predominantly solid (Fig. 5). Surgery was performed via a right frontotemporal craniotomy. After exposure of the

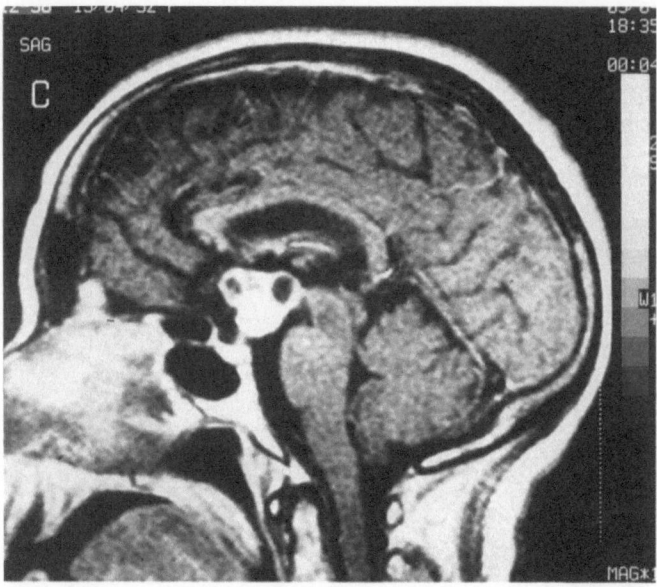

Fig. 2. Case 1: preoperative, contrast-enhanced cerebral MRI showing a supraretro-sellar tumor with solid and cystic components

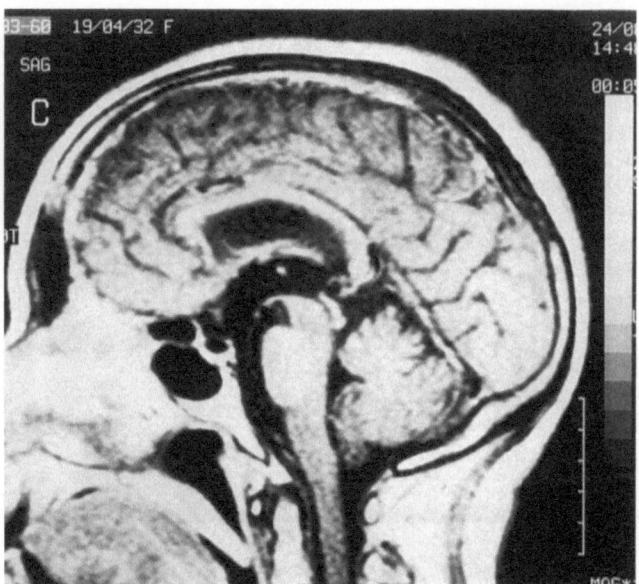

Fig. 3. Case 1: postoperative, contrast-enhanced cerebral MRI, demonstrating total removal of the craniopharyngioma (compare with Fig. 2)

chiasmatic region and opening of the sylvian fissure, the chiasm appeared completely prefixed: the lamina terminalis was markedly swollen by the tumor. The craniopharyngioma was totally removed, mostly through the lamina terminalis. Resection of the retrochiasmatic portion of the tumor made it

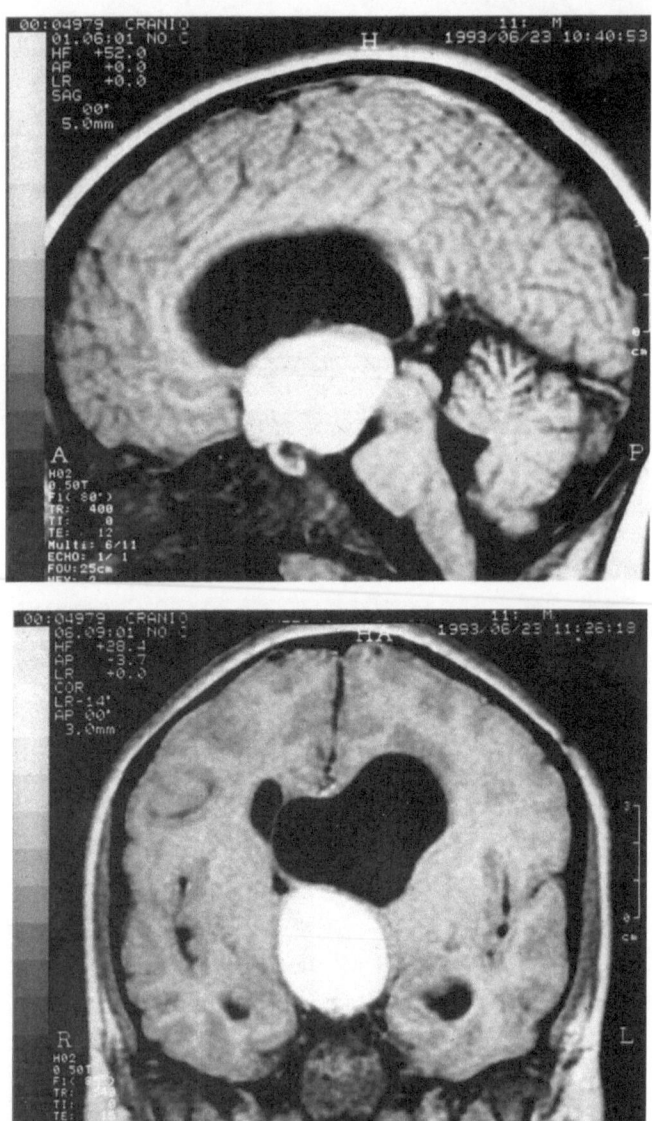

Fig. 4. Case 2: preoperative, contrast-enhanced cerebral MRI. *Top*, sagittal view; *bottom*, coronal view

clear that the chiasm was not completely prefixed, but was pushed forward by the tumor itself; in fact, it was possible to divide the pituitary stalk, invaded by the tumor, through the reappeared interoptic space.

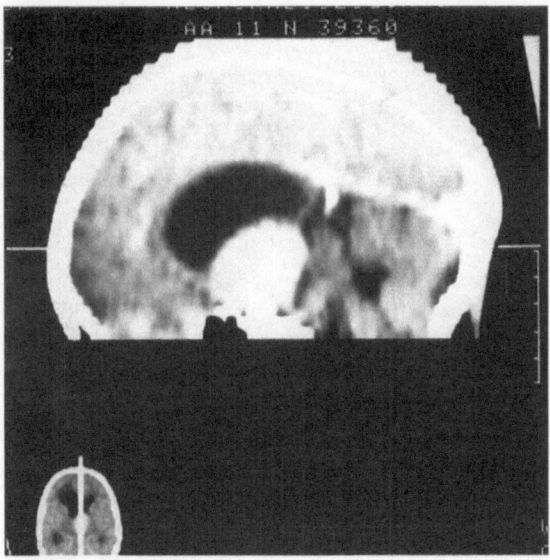

Fig. 5. Case 2: sagittal, reformatted, contrast-enhanced CT scan demonstrating that the tumor is predominantly solid

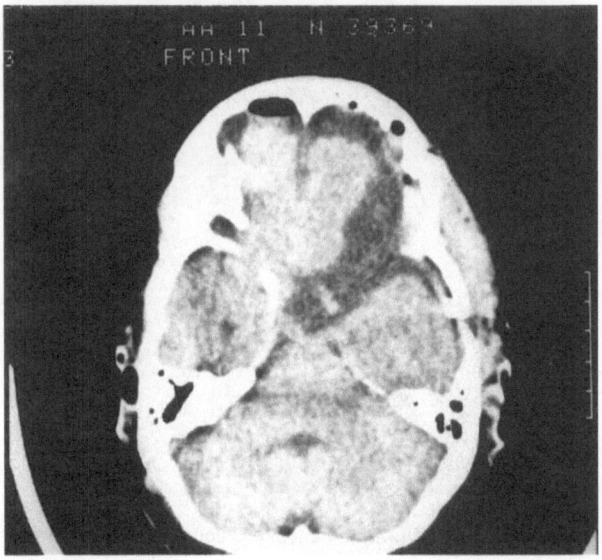

Fig. 6. Case 2: non-enhanced, axial CT scan the day after surgery, demonstrating the wide opening of the sylvian fissure

A CT scan performed the day after surgery showed the wide opening of the sylvian fissure (Fig. 6). Postoperative, contrast-enhanced MRI confirmed total removal of the craniopharyngioma (Fig. 7). Moreover, a remarkable

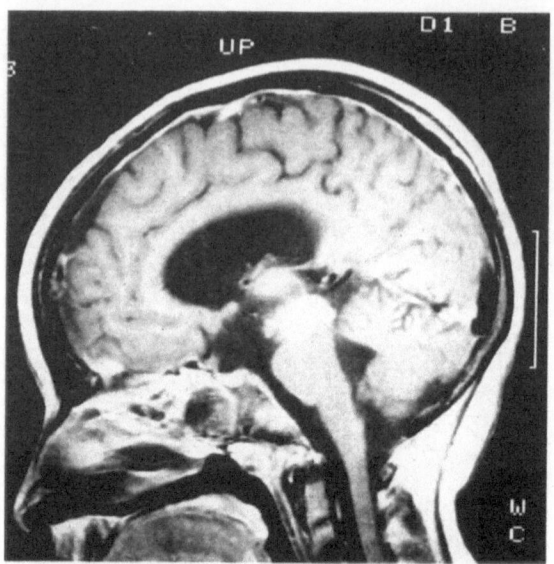

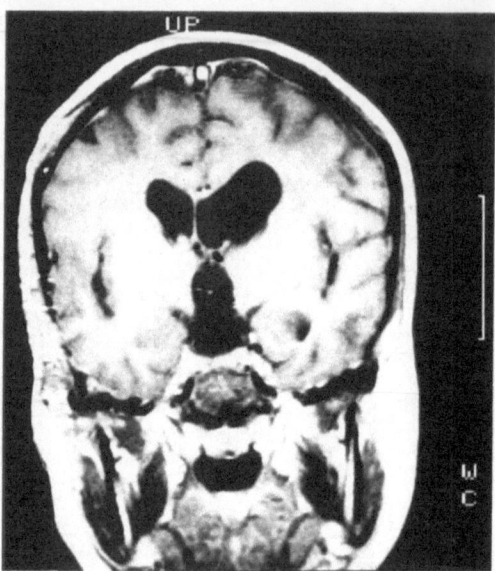

Fig. 7. Case 2: postoperative, contrast-enhanced cerebral MRI, demonstrating complete removal of craniopharyngioma. *Top*, sagittal view; *bottom*, coronal view (compare with Fig. 4). The decrease in left ventricular size was achieved without any ventricular shunting

decrease of left ventricular size was evident, achieved without any ventricular shunting.

Conclusions

In our experience, the technique used allowed adequate exposure and removal of most craniopharyngiomas, with low morbidity. Moreover, the slight unilateral frontal lobe retraction prevented the occurrence of serious bifrontal damage and bilateral avulsion of olfactory nerves.

References

Backlund EO (1973a) Studies on craniopharyngiomas. III. Stereotaxic treatment with intracystic Yttrium-90. Acta Chir Scand 139:237-247

Backlund EO (1973b) Studies on craniopharyngiomas. IV. Stereotaxic treatment with radiosurgery. Acta Chir Scand 139:344-351

Backlund EO (1988) Colloidal radioisotopes as part of a multimodality treatment of craniopharyngiomas. J Neurosurg Sci 33:95-97

Backlund EO, Johansson L, Sarby B (1972) Studies on craniopharyngiomas II. Treatment by stereotaxis and radiosurgery. Acta Chir Scand 138:749-759

Baskin DS, Wilson CB (1986) Surgical management of craniopharyngiomas: a review of 74 cases. J Neurosurg 65:22-27

Bond WH, Richards D, Turner E (1965) Experiences with radioactive gold in the treatment of craniopharyngioma. J Neurol Neurosurg Psychiatry 28:30-38

Broggi G, Giorgi C, Franzini A, Servello D, Solero CL (1988) Preliminary results of intracavitary treatment of craniopharyngioma with bleomycin. J Neurosurg Sci 33:145- 148

Carmel PW, Antunes JL, Chang CH (1982) Craniopharyngiomas in children. Neurosurgery 11:382-389

Colombo F, Benedetti A, Pozza F, Avanzo RC, Marchetti C, Chierego G, Zanardo A (1985) External stereotactic irradiation by linear accelerator. Neurosurgery 16:154-160

Fisher E, Welch K, Belli JA, Wallan J, Shillito JJ, Winston KR, Cassady R (1985) Treatment of craniopharyngiomas in children: 1972-1981. J Neurosurg 62:496-501

Guidetti B, Fraioli B (1979) Craniopharyngiomas. Results of surgical treatment. Acta Neurochir Suppl (Wien) 28:349-351

Hoffman HJ, Hendrick EB, Humphreys RP, Buncic JR, Armstrong DL, Jenkin RDT (1977) Management of craniopharyngiomas in children. J Neurosurg 47:218-227

Julow J, Lanyi F, Hajda M, Simkovics M, Aramy I, Toth S, Pasztor E (1985) The radiotherapy of cystic craniopharyngioma with intracystic installation of Yttrium-90 silicate colloid. Acta Neurochir (Wien) 74:94-99

Katz EL (1975) Late results of radical excision of craniopharyngiomas in children. J Neurosurg 42:86-90

Kobayashi T, Kageyama N, Ohara K (1981) Internal irradiation for cystic craniopharyngioma. J Neurosurg 55:896-903

Lapras C, Patet JD, Mottolese C, Gharbi S, Lapras C Jr (1987) Craniopharyngiomas in childhood: analysis of 42 cases. Progr Exp Tumor Res 30:350-358

Leksell L (1983) Stereotactic radiosurgery. J Neurol Neurosurg Psychiatry 46:797-803

Leksell L, Backlund EO, Johansson L (1967) Treatment of craniopharyngiomas. Acta Chir Scand 133:345-350

Manaka S, Teramoto A, Takakura K (1985) The efficacy of radiotherapy for craniopharyngioma. J Neurosurg 62:648-656

Munari C, Landre E, Musolino A, Turak B, Habert MO, Chodkiewicz JP (1988) Long term results of stereotactic endocavitary beta irradiation of craniopharyngioma cysts. J Neurosurg Sci 33:99-105

Mundinger F, Hoefer T (1974) Protracted long term irradiation of inoperable midbrain tumors by stereotactic Curie-therapy using Iridium 192. Acta Neurochir Suppl (Wien) 21:93-100

Pang D (1993) Surgical management of craniopharyngioma. In: Sekhar LN, Janecka IP (eds) Surgery of cranial base tumors. Raven, New York, pp 787-807

Pollack IF, Lunsford LD, Slamovitis IL, Gumermann LW, Levine G, Robinson AG (1988) Stereotactic intracavitary irradiation for cystic craniopharyngiomas. J Neurosurg 68:227-233

Richmond IL, Wara WM, Wilson CB (1980) Role of radiation therapy in the management of craniopharyngioma in children. Neurosurgery 6:513-517

Shapiro K, Till K, Grant ND (1979) Craniopharyngiomas in childhood. A rational approach to treatment. J Neurosurg 50:617-623

Spaziante R, de Divitiis E, Irace C, Cappabianca P, Caputi F (1989) Management of primary or recurring grossly cystic craniopharyngiomas by means of draining systems. Topic review and 6 case reports. Acta Neurochir (Wien) 97:95-106

Strauss L, Sturn V, Georgi P, Schlegel W, Ostertag H, Clorins JH, van Kaick G (1982) Radioisotope therapy for cystic craniopharyngiomas. Int J Radiat Oncol Biol Phys 8:1581-1585

Sweet WH (1976) Radical surgical treatment of craniopharyngioma. Clin Neurosurg 23:52-79

Symon L, Sprich W (1985) Radical excision of craniopharyngioma. Results in 20 patients. J Neurosurg 62:174-181

Takahashi H, Nazakawa, Shimura T (1985) Evaluation of postoperative intratumoral injection of bleomycin for craniopharyngioma in children. J Neurosurg 62:120-127

Valentino V (1988) Radiosurgery in cerebral tumors and AVM. Acta Neurochir Suppl (Wien) 42:193-197

Viramuthu N, Benton TF (1983) The management of craniopharyngiomas. Clin Radiol 34:629-632

Yasargil MG, Curcic M, Kis M, Siegenthaler G, Teddy PJ, Roth P (1990) Total removal of craniopharyngiomas: approaches and long term results in 144 patients. J Neurosurg 73:3-11

Therapeutic Role of Intracavitary Bleomycin Administration in Cystic Craniopharyngioma

G. Broggi*, C. Giorgi*, A. Franzini*, F. Leocata*, and D. Riva

Introduction

Craniopharyngioma is a histologically benign tumor which can be totally cured by radical surgical removal; however, such a result can only be achieved in a limited percentage of patients. The presence of delicate, highly functional structures surrounding the area where the tumor is commonly located makes total removal very difficult when the tumor is adherent to these structures. Children are particularly exposed to the effect of damage to the hypothalamus and because of this a conservative surgical attitude is frequently adopted that often results in tumor regrowth.

As a consequence, a number of alternatives have been proposed to treat tumors that cannot be totally removed safely. Radiotherapy has been most commonly advocated, normally in association with surgery; more recently, though, a stereotactic radiosurgery has been proposed in which a highly focused single dose is administered (Backlund et al. 1972).

If cysts are a prominent feature surgical alternatives to the tumor removal are available, especially in childhood. Intracavitary treatment (Backlund 1979) using isotopes or bleomycin (Takahashi et al. 1985; Broggi et al. 1989) has been proposed to control or delay the growth of cysts, in order to postpone surgery until it is required because of the increase in the solid portion of the tumor. The rationale of this treatment derives from cell kinetics data obtained in these tumors (Broggi et al. 1994).

In this paper we present our experience with intracavitary bleomycin treatment, performed in patients in whom symptoms were sustained by the growth of the cystic portion of a craniopharyngioma, in order to control the risks of hormonal deficiency in younger patients, and to avoid or delay surgery in adults in cases of solitary cysts, largely prevailing in the solid portion.

Istituto Nazionale Neurologico "C. Besta", Via Celoria 11, 20133 Milan, Italy
* Div. Neurosurgery
  Div. Pediatric Neurology

Materials and Method

From 1986 to date, we have used intracystic bleomycin to treat 19 patients in whom craniopharyngioma had a prominent cystic component. Almost invariably this treatment has been later complemented with surgical removal. The aim of this study is to evaluate the efficacy of the procedure on the cyst treated. Clinical and neuroradiological long-term follow-up data are only available for14 patients, who are the subjects of this report.

The clinical material is summarized in Table 1. There were seven patients (three boys, four girls) aged between 3 and 12 years and seven (four men, three women) aged between 26 and 65 years.

Symptoms in four patients in both groups were sustained by the cysts,

Table 1. Clinical manifestations of craniopharyngioma cysts (14 of 19 treated patients)

Patient	Age (years)	Sex	Location	Symptoms	Previous surgery	Hydro-cephalus
1	12	F	Suprasellar	Field defect, short stature	No	No
2	9	M	Intrasuprasellar	Headache	Shunt	Yes
3	7	F	Intrasuprasellar	Field defect, DI	No	No
4	8	M	Intrasuprasellar	Field defect	Yes	No
5	3	F	Intrasuprasellar	Field defect	No	No
6	11	F	Intrasuprasellar	Field defect, DI growth deficiency	Yes	No
7	6	M	Prepontine	Headache	Yes	No
8	30	M	Supraretrosellar	Headache, field defect	Yes	Yes
9	26	M	Suprasellar	Field defect	No	No
10	45	F	Suprasellar	Field defect, memory impairment, DI	No	No
11	52	M	Suprasellar	Headache field defect	No	Yes
12	46	F	Suprasellar	Field defect, DI	No	Yes
13	65	F	Suprasellar	Field defect	Yes	No
14	34	M	Intrasuprasellar	Field defect	Yes	No

F, female; M, male; DI, diabetes insipidus

consisting in visual field defects, hormone deficiency, or signs of increased intracranial pressure. One patient (no. 2) had received a shunt prior to admission to our hospital; two others patients (nos. 8 and 11) had ventricular enlargement that did not require shunting: cyst drainage restored CSF circulation.

Cyst location was almost invariably intra-and suprasellar, even in patients who had previously been operated upon, with the exception of patients 7 and 8, in whom the cyst had developed in the retrosellar-prepontine region.

All patients treated received bleomycin via a stereotactically positioned intracystic catheter. Starting in1987 a computer-assisted procedure developed at our institution was introduced to assist the surgeon in selecting a trajectory of approach avoiding the passage through the ventricular system or the subarachnoid space, while choosing a convenient location for the catheter tip in the center of the cyst (Fig. 1; Giorgi et al. 1987). Bleomycin was administered at 48-h intervals over a period of 3 - 30 days in quantities ranging from 3 to 42 mg. Drug administration followed the aspiration of a variable amount of cystic content, according to the initial cystic volume and the appearance of fluid. Single doses ranged from 1.5 to 5 mg. Five patients required multiple administration cycles (2 - 4) up to 55 mg total bleomycin. No toxic effects have been reported apart from fever and headache often occurring the day following the administration and occasional, short-term

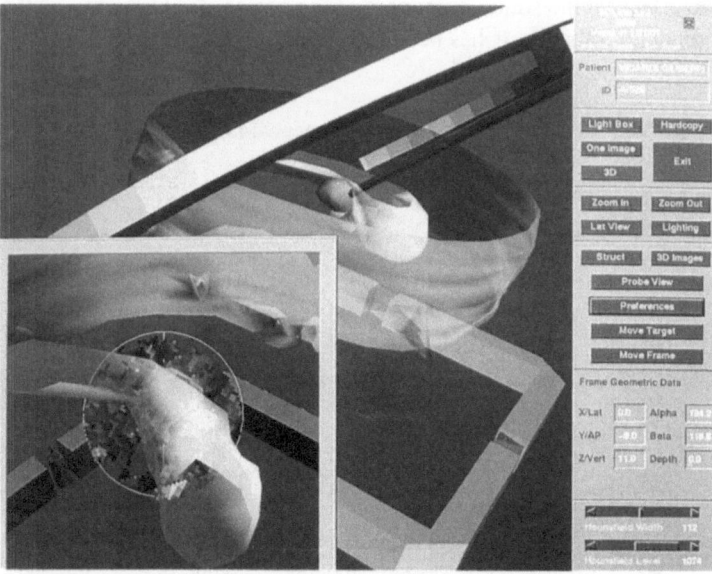

Fig. 1. Three-dimensional reconstruction of craniopharyngioma cyst, lateral ventricle and probe trajectory, in stereotactic space. *Insert* at *lower left* shows probe's eye view, with ventricle crossed by the trajectory

nausea and vomiting. A complication worth noting occurred in patient 12, in whom a single administration of 5 mg of bleomycin was followed by bilateral hypoacusia which developed in a few days. There is no explanation for such an acute complication that is related to the drug since communication with the CSF compartment has been demonstrated only in that patient. One other patient had an ischemic attack involving the ipsilateral middle cerebral artery territory 3 months after the last administration of bleomycin.

Lactate dehydrogenase (LDH) activity was measured daily in the cystic fluid; a remarkable increase in the activity of this enzyme was noted in all cases immediately after the onset of therapy (four to ten times the baseline value), followed by a slow decrease. No definite pattern of LDH behavior has been found to predict the treatment efficacy.

Treated cysts disappeared in eight patients and reduced in size and stabilized in all others. Follow-up times range from 2 months for patient 10, followed by subtotal surgical removal of the solid component which was responsible for the persisting field defect, to 7 years in patients 3, 4, and 7, never operated on after this treatment. All other patients underwent partial, subtotal, or total removal of the solid portion of the craniopharyngioma within a period ranging from 11 months to 7 years (Table 2). At operation, no abnormalities were found, with the exception of the frequent finding of a "thick membrane" surrounding the implanted catheter, probably the result of a fibrotic effect of the treatment (Fig. 2).

No effect on the solid component of the tumor, nor influence on the development of other cysts has been recorded.

Table 2. Clinical outcome of bleomycin treatment (14 of 19 treated patients)

Patient	Bleomycin/ cycle (mg)	Cycles	Follow-up	Cyst	Surgery
1	5	1	7 years	Disappeared	Partial
2	3	1	13 months	Disappeared	Total
3	24, 25, 15, 10	4	7 years	Reduced	No
4	12, 25	2	7 years	Reduced	No
5	24	1	5 years	Disappeared	Total
6	15	1	2 years	Reduced	Partial
7	42, 2, 1.5	3	7 years	Disappeared	No
8	25, 10, 25	3	11 months	Disappeared	Total
9	25	1	3 years	Disappeared	Subtotal
10	10	1	2 months	Disappeared	Subtotal
11	40	1	1 year, 9 months	Reduced	Subtotal
12	5	1	1 year	Reduced	Subtotal
13	3, 3, 1	3	5 years	Reduced	Subtotal
14	15	1	1 year, 10 months	Reduced	Partial

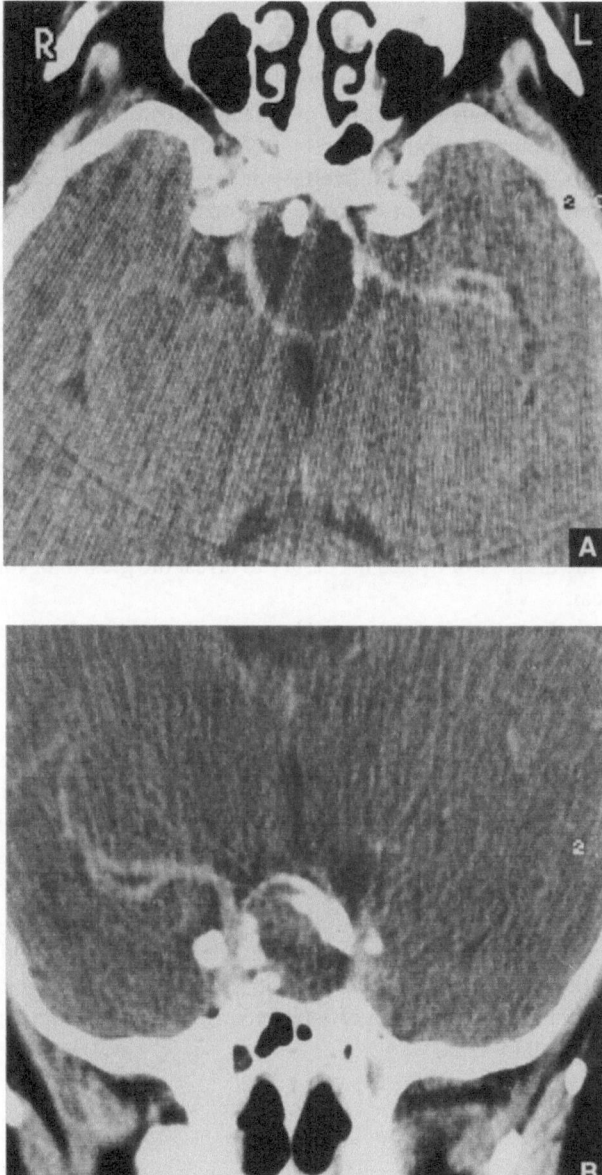

Fig. 2 A, B. Patient before (**A**) and after (**B**) bleomycin treatment (1-year follow-up). Cyst size unchanged until surgical removal of growing solid component 5 years later. Note calcification which developed on cystic wall

Discussion

As previously reported (Takahashi et al. 1985; Broggi et al. 1989), intracavitary bleomycin treatment is an effective means of controlling cystic components of craniopharyngiomas, whereby toxic effects have been recorded in about 10% of patients. Bilateral hypoacusia, recorded in patient 12, with an onset closely related to the treatment, was possibly due to its direct toxic effect, since CSF was obtained by aspiration from the reservoir on the day following a single bleomycin administration (5 mg). The ischemic lesion which occurred in the second patient may have been mediated by vasospasm secondary to bleomycin leakage in the middle artery cistern. A single administration has nevertheless been sufficient to control the cyst's size for 1 year. Surgery then became necessary, due to the increase in the solid portion of the tumor.

In all other patients the control of the cyst's size was obtained with a single or multiple (up to four) cycles of drug administration; no correlation has been found between the cyst's initial volume or LDH values during treatment and the number of cycles necessary to arrest the growth or for the cyst to disappear.

Although the available data cannot be used to establish a treatment protocol relating patient's age, cyst size, tumor type, and LDH values to the dose and number of treatment cycles, we consider intracavitary bleomycin administration a valid therapeutic alternative to open surgery in the management of cystic craniopharyngiomas. In patients in whom symptoms are sustained by a single cyst, effective control of its volume can be obtained with this drug without side effects if the intracavitary catheter is carefully positioned and if the cyst is tightly isolated from basal cisternal spaces so as to avoid major complications due to the local toxic effect of bleomycin on cranial nerves and vessels.

This result is of particular relevance in the treatment of children with symptomatic cystic craniopharyngioma: in these cases bleomycin treatment can delay operation, offering an efficient control over the symptoms related to the cyst's volume.

References

Backlund (1979) Stereotactic radiosurgery in intracranial tumors and vascular malformations. In: Krayenbuhl H (ed) Advances and technical standards in neurosurgery. Springer, Vienna New York, p 88

Backlund EO, Johanson L, Sarby B (1972) Studies on craniopharyngiomas. II. Treatment by stereotactic radiosurgery. Acta Chir Scand 138:749-759

Broggi G, Giorgi C, Franzini A, Servello D, Solero CL (1989) Preliminary results of intracavitary treatment of craniopharyngioma with bleomycin. J Neurol Sci 33:145-148

Broggi G, Franzini A, Cajola L, Pluchino F (1994) Cell kinetic investigations in craniopharyngioma: preliminary results and considerations. Pediatr Neurosurg 2151:21-23

Giorgi C, Ongania E, Franzini A, Broggi G (1987) Three dimensional reconstruction of neuroradiological data within a stereotactic frame of reference for surgery of visible targets. Appl Neurophysiol 50:77-80

Takahashi H, Nakazawa S, Shimura T (1985) Evaluation of postoperative intratumoral injection of bleomycin for craniopharyngioma in children. J Neurosurg 62:120-127

Gamma Knife Radiosurgery and Intracystic Colloidal Isotope Treatment of Craniopharyngiomas

T. Rähn

Introduction

Stereotactic treatment of craniopharyngiomas was developed in the 1960s in our department as a minimally invasive alternative to conventional large craniotomy with attempts to radically extirpate the tumor (Backlund et al. 1972; Backlund 1973a, 1973b; Bosch and Beekhuis 1979; Julow et al. 1985). Before the complete development of microsurgery as it is known today major surgical interventions were often accompanied by postoperative complications and dramatic intensive care, with a high risk of mortality and morbidity. Consequently, it was a great step forward to be able to control these tumors by stereotactic procedures, which can be carried out under local anesthesia and the patient released from the hospital the following day. With stereotactic treatment the tumor is not extirpated, but in the long term, the tumor remnant has been quiescent in many cases and offered the patient a possibility to maintain a good quality of life.

The development of microsurgery with modern techniques including ultrasonic disintegration and lasers as well as the increasing skill of microsurgeons, however, has made it possible to radically remove many of the tumors previously regarded as very difficult. Other presentations during this workshop have demonstrated excellent results with these modern techniques. However, there still remains a small group of craniopharyngiomas that are not radically removed and hence need additional treatment. We have also seen recurrences after "radical extirpations" with one or several large cysts with extremely thin cyst walls, which are difficult to dissect completely at reoperation. This selected group of craniopharyngiomas can be treated by stereotactic procedures such as intracavitary isotope treatment of cystic portions with colloid, pure β-emitting ^{90}Y and for small solid portions Gamma Knife surgery. The use of stereotactic high quality magnetic resonance imaging (MRI) has tremendously improved the anatomical information, so that at Gamma Knife surgery critical surrounding cranial nerves can be avoided and more patients can now be accepted for radiosurgery.

Department of Neurosurgery, Karolinska Hospital, S-104 01 Stockholm, Sweden

The cost-benefit of stereotactic procedures is important since a patient who receives stereotactic puncture with intracystic colloid isotope treatment only needs overnight hospitalization and Gamma Knife surgery can be performed as a single procedure on an outpatient basis.

Patients

As craniopharyngiomas are extremely rare most of the patients treated at Karolinska Hospital are referred from abroad, which presents great difficulty in classifying the wide range of previous microsurgery conducted by various neurosurgeons and the varying nature of the tumors as to the proportion of solid and cystic components. Several attempts have been made to trace these cases, without success. However, in order to assess the long-term outcome of this treatment, in 1989 my tutor E.O. Backlund and I, in cooperation with Dr Norén, endocrinologists, radiologists, and ophthalmologists, published the long-term results of 42 consecutive Swedish patients from 1964 to 1976 with previously untreated craniopharyngiomas that were followed for 10-23 years until 1987 (Backlund et al. 1989). The patients were categorized into three groups, those having predominantly cystic lesions (24), those with polycystic tumors with an appreciable solid portion (11), and those with fairly small, predominantly solid tumors (7). As a rule the first two groups could be given intracavitary treatment with ^{90}Y in a colloidal solution. For the entirely solid tumors Gamma Knife radiosurgery was used as a first choice.

Twenty-five patients were treated exclusively with stereotactic methods, intracavitary colloid isotope irradiation of cysts, and/or Gamma Knife radiosurgery. In another five, initially treated by stereotactic methods, further treatment was considered necessary and they additionally underwent open surgical removal (four cases) and conventional radiotherapy (one case), respectively. In the remaining 12 the first choice was surgical removal (nine cases), radiotherapy (one case), and a combination of these two modalities in two patients. In this group of nonstereotactically treated, five tumors were very large and had a large number of small cysts and large solid portions. Six patients had, at stereotactic explorative puncture, cyst contents so rich in cholesterol that the porridge-like substance was impossible to aspirate or mix with colloid ^{90}Y and hence the tumor and cyst were removed using open surgery.

Results

Of the 25 patients treated exclusively with stereotactic methods four died of intercurrent diseases, three revealed at autopsy no recurrent tumor, and the fourth had a very small remnant of the suprasellar cyst.

Computed tomography (CT) follow-up in the remaining 21 patients demonstrated in the monocystic group 13 patients with collapsed cyst remnants and one with marked reduction of the initial cyst. In the multicystic group none of the four patients had expanding lesions and in the third group of those with entirely solid tumors the three patients had only insignificant tumor remnants.

Hence the ^{90}Y injection as a rule caused a pronounced and permanent shrinkage of the tumor cyst, in many cases virtually a radiological disappearance, combined with an opening of the cisterns around the tumor. The shrinkage was gradual and as a rule not complete until after many months. Occasionally, the decrease in cyst size after ^{90}Y injection was slower than expected and a repuncture with a mere aspiration of the contents was performed, initiating definite and complete collapse of the cyst.

Out of 29 eyes in patients with preoperative visual field defects at follow-up four had normal fields, another four were unchanged, 13 were improved, and eight were worse. Very often the improvement of visual acuity and fields is prompt at the puncture - the patient under local anesthesia reports a momentary dramatic regain of vision. In one patient with seriously impaired vision on first admission, only finger-counting left, vision was completely regained after ^{90}Y treatment, but 9 months later she was readmitted because of rapid deterioration of the vision in the same (left) eye. A microsurgical exploration was performed with no finding of tumor. The suprasellar cistern was free from adherences. The optic pathways were without gross changes except a small translucent area in the left optic nerve, most probably an infarction secondary to thrombosis of one of the supplying tiny arteries maybe caused by stretching of the artery when the cyst collapsed. Another patient experienced fairly sudden diplopia 9 days after ^{90}Y instillation due to palsy of the third cranial nerve. As a noxious effect of the yttrium was suspected, the cyst was repunctured and the contents aspirated, but this made the oculomotor palsy worse. Apparently, the cyst capsule had a preexisting attachment to the third cranial nerve that was stretched when the cyst collapsed. Nine years later oculomotor nerve paresis in this patient was almost absent. The former case as well as the striking feature of follow-up radiological examination with the persistence of open cisterns and spacious conditions around collapsed cysts verifies that intracystic short-range β-irradiation from ^{90}Y isotope does not induce adhesions or scarring in the vicinity of the cyst and thus does not make later attempts at microsurgical dissection more difficult. Hence, it could be stated that, contrary to what is claimed, stereotactic treatment as the first choice might even facilitate later open surgery, should it become necessary.

At follow-up at the department of endocrinology the study was not focused exclusively on the 25 stereotactically treated patients. Eight of the nine surviving patients primarily operated with surgical removal, and two patients surviving after initial stereotactic treatment followed by open surgical removal were included (Sääf et al. 1989). In total, 31 patients were followed. Of 31 patients 20 (65%) had subjectively no or only minor disturbances of their everyday life because of the tumor disease. Five of 31 (16%) had headache, visual disturbance, or psychiatric disturbance. Of the patients 22 (71%) had subjectively good memory function, 58% had a driver's license, three of them even a pilot's license or a license for driving a bus or truck.

Most patients adapted well to their social situation. Of the 29 patients 23 (79%) below the age of 65 were in regular work; 21 (72%) worked full-time; the two remaining female patients had small children and worked part-time outside the home. Only three of the patients had university education, while heavy farm work, truck driving, directing a large company, and anesthesia nursing were some of the more demanding occupations represented.

Four of the patients had a disability pension. Two treated at an early age (6 and 15 years) had intellectual and neurological handicaps, but had also had complementary open surgery. The third patient, formerly a hospital secretary, stereotactically treated for a cyst only had a subjectively very disabling headache, but she managed to start up a dog kennel. Another woman had had a disability pension since the age of 58 because of undiagnosed panhypopituitarism. These two women are living independent lives.

In this study the "disability rate" was found to be 14%, compared to 4%-8% in the overall Swedish population in 1984. This figure is low when compared to other studies in which 17%-60% had major complications following surgery or were "not able to care for themselves" (Amendola et al. 1985; Mori et al. 1980; Symon and Sprich 1985; Thomsett et al. 1980). Decreased sociability and psychological deficits have been found when young patients with craniopharyngiomas have been treated with open neurosurgery and radiation therapy (Clopper et al. 1977; Galatzer et al. 1981; Lapras et al 1987), but also among patients with pituitary deficiency of other origin (Galatzer et al. 1987; Lindqvist 1966). The reasons for this might be a complex of psychosocial sequela and possible organic brain syndromes induced by the tumor or its surgical treatment. In several studies the patients are found to have behavioral and psychological disturbances but normal IQ (Clopper et al. 1977; Danoff et al. 1983; Flick and Michel 1986; Galatzer et al. 1981; Lapras et al 1987). Some investigators have found evidence for frontal lobe dysfunction in patients operated upon by the subfrontal route (Cavazutti et al. 1983; Stelling et al. 1986).

Hence, the result of the study argues for an individualized treatment program in the management of craniopharyngiomas, including the atraumatic stereotactic treatment modality as an important alternative and in some cases as the first choice. The patients will then be found to have a lower long-term tumor-related mortality, shorter hospitalization, and higher rates of working capacity.

References

Amendola BE, Gebarski SS, Bermudez AG (1985) Analysis of treatment results in craniopharyngioma. J Clin Oncol 3:252-258

Backlund EO (1973a) Studies on craniopharyngiomas III. Stereotaxic treatment with intracystic yttrium-90. Acta Chir Scand 139:237-247

Backlund EO (1973b) Studies on craniopharyngiomas IV. Stereotaxic treatment with radiosurgery. Acta Chir Scand 139:344-351

Backlund EO, Johansson L, Sarby B (1972) Studies on craniopharyngiomas II. Treatment by stereotaxis and radiosurgery. Acta Chir Scand 138:749-759

Backlund EO, Axelsson B, Bergstrand CG, Eriksson A-L, Norén G, Ribbesjö E, Rähn T, Schnell PO, Tallstedt L, Sääf M, Thorén M (1989) Treatment of craniopharyngiomas – the stereotactic approach in a ten to twenty-three years' perspective. I. Surgical, radiological and ophthalmological aspects. Acta Neurochir (Wien) 99:11-19

Bosch DA, Beekhuis H (1979) Stereotactic application of ^{90}Yttrium in cystic brain tumors. Neuropädiatrie 10:414-415

Cavazutti V, Fischer EG, Welch K, Belli JA, Winston KR (1983) Neurological and psychophysiological sequelae following treatment of craniopharyngioma in children. J Neurosurg 59:409-417

Clopper RR, Meyer WJ, Udvarhelyi GB, Money J, Aarabi B, Mulvihill JJ, Piasio M (1977) Postsurgical IQ and behavioral data on twenty patients with a history of childhood craniopharyngioma. Psychoneuroendocrinology 2:365-377

Danoff BF, Cowchock FS, Kramer S (1983) Childhood craniopharyngioma: survival, local control, endocrine and neurologic function following radiotherapy. Int J Radiat Oncol Biol Phys 9:171-175

Flick TH, Michel M (1986) Rehabilitation jugendlicher Kraniopharyngeom-Patienten. Rehabilitation 25:45-52

Galatzer A, Nofar E, Beit-Halachmi N, Aran O, Shalit M, Roitman A, Laron Z (1981) Intellectual and psychosocial functions in children, adolescents and young adults before and after operation for craniopharyngioma. Child Care Health Dev 7:307-316

Galatzer A, Aran O, Beit-Halachmi N, Nofar E, Rubitchek J, Pertzelan A, Laron Z (1987) The impact of long-term therapy by a multi-disciplinary team on the education, occupation and marital status of growth hormone deficient patients after termination of therapy. Clin Endocrinol 27:191-196

Julow J, Lanyi F, Hajda M, et al (1985) The radiotherapy of cystic craniopharyngiomas with intracystic instillation of ^{90}Y silicate colloid. Acta Neurochir (Wien) 74:94-99

Lapras C, Patet JD, Mottolese C, Gharbi S, Lapras Ch (1987) Craniopharyngiomas in childhood: analysis of 42 cases. Prog Exp Tumor Res 30:350-358

Lindqvist G (1966) Mental changes after transsphenoidal hypophysectomy. Acta Phsychiatr Scand Suppl 42:190

Mori K, Handa H, Murata T, Takeuchi T, Miwa S, Osaka K (1980) Results of treatment of craniopharyngioma. Childs Brain 6:303-312

Stelling MW, McKay SE, Carr WA, Walsh JW, Baumann RJ (1986) Frontal lobe lesions and cognitive function in craniopharyngioma survivors. Am J Dis Child 140:710-714

Symon L, Sprich W (1985) Radical excision of craniopharyngioma. Results in 20 patients. J Neurosurg 62:174-181

Sääf M, Thorén M, Bergstrand CG, Norén G, Rähn T, Tallstedt L, Backlund EO (1989) Treatment of craniopharyngiomas – the stereotactic approach in a ten to twenty-three years perspective. II. Psychosocial situation and pituitary function. Acta Neurochir (Wien) 99:97-103

Thomsett MJ, Conte FA, Kaplan SL, Grumbach MM (1980) Endocrine and neurologic outcome in childhood craniopharyngioma: Review of effect of treatment in 42 patients. J Pediatr 97:728-735

Three-Dimensional Dosimetry for LINAC-Based Radiosurgery and Fractionated Stereotactic Radiotherapy of Craniopharyngiomas

C. Giorgi, M. Luzzara, U. Cerchiari*, and A. Gramaglia*

Introduction

Stereotactic radiosurgery performed with the Gamma Unit (Leksell 1983) or LINACs (Colombo et al. 1985) and heavy-charged particles beams (Kjellberg et al. 1983) has become a part of the neurosurgical armamentarium and is being met with growing interest at an increasing number of neurosurgical centers worldwide. Introduced by Leksell (1951) as a method of delivery of ionizing radiation energy to destroy a target volume of living tissue (healthy and/or pathologic) without causing radiation damage to the adjacent tissues, it has evolved from the treatment of functional disorders of the brain to an alternative to open surgery for arteriovenous malformations, neurinomas, pinealomas, pituitary tumors, and craniopharyngiomas (Steiner and Lindguist 1987; Betti et al. 1989; Noren 1983; Backlund 1972a, 1972b).

All available equipment fulfills the criteria for delivering the dose with sufficient precision in terms of amount of energy and spatial distribution, with a steep dose drop-off outside the target volume. All systems use stereotactic frames for calculating the treatment geometry and for dose targeting during treatment.

In this paper we present a dose-planning system developed at the Istituto Neurologico, Milan, Italy, that makes it possible to treat suitable lesions with the spatial accuracy delivered by modern neuroimaging techniques. The planning system has been designed for use with linear accelerators fitted with sets of collimators and frame fixation devices, which allow the precise distribution of the planned dose during treatment (Fig. 1).

Div Neurosurgery, Istituto Nazionale Neurologico "C. Besta", Via Celoria 11, 20133 Milan, Italy
* Div. Radiotherapy, Istituto Nazionale dei Tumori, Via Venezian 11, 20133 Milan, Italy

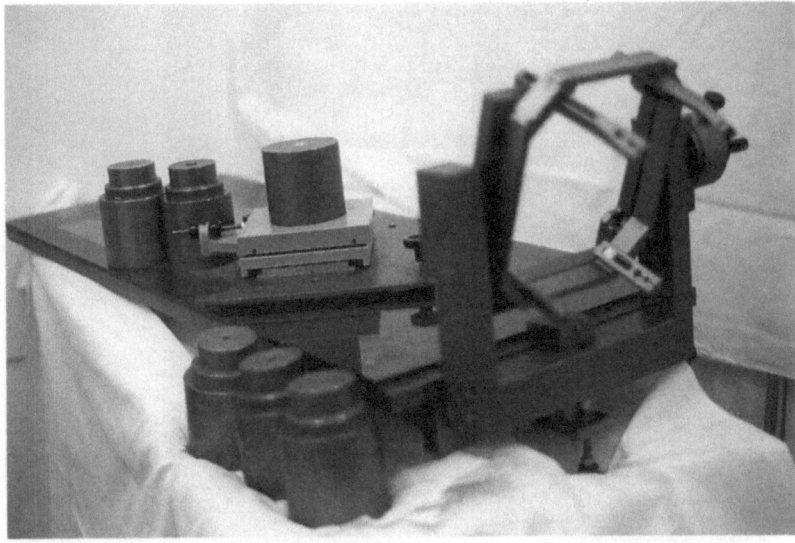

Fig. 1. Synoptic view of the stereotactic LINAC accessories: A set of collimators of various diameters (on an x, y micrometric accelerator-head mount) and a frame holder of the couch-mounted type can be seen

Materials and Methods

The planning system was developed on a dedicated graphic workstation, with an adequate CPU for fast three-dimensional calculation of the isodose distribution and effective rendering of graphics, obtained with a graphic accelerator, capable of the displaying 10 000 shaded polygons per second.

Images are transferred from the diagnostic consoles of computed tomographic (CT) or magnetic resonance imaging (MRI) equipment to the graphic computer by means of an 8-inch magnetic tape. Image formats are converted into the ACR-NEMA standard.

Image manipulation routines allow the identification and manual contouring of the lesion and of healthy structures, whose position is relevant for treatment planning. Linear interpolation algorithms display three-dimensional structures with a shaded surface-rendering technique. Automatic contouring algorithms are used to define the head volume within the stereotactic space so as to calculate the dose absorption along each arc. The stereotactic space is defined with a semiautomatic procedure that recognizes the location of the localizer's artifacts on each image (Fig. 2).

A set of utilities can be used in this phase to look for image distortion and to disclose calibration errors.

Treatment geometry is planned on the stereotactically defined anatomy. The collimator's diameter is selected and the number and position of arcs defined. Normally, a nine-arc technique is implemented (Fig. 3).

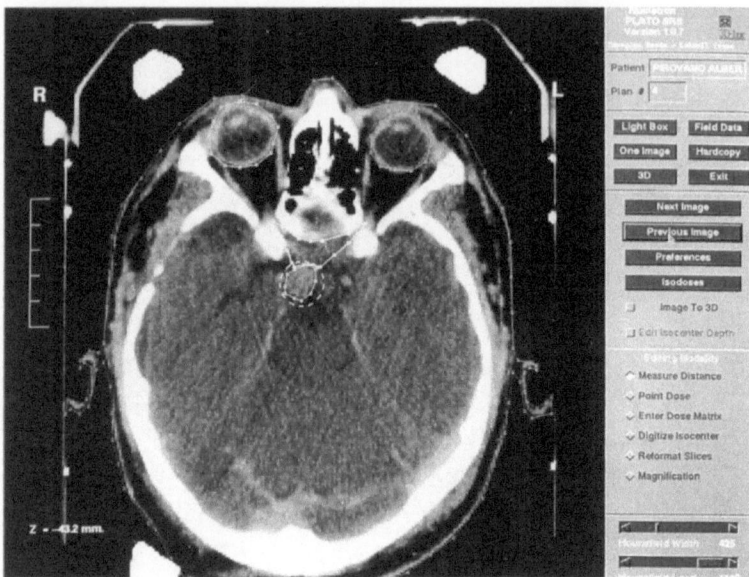

Fig. 2. CT image, with localizer's artifacts surrounding head. Automatic and semiautomatic procedures identify the image plane, based on the positions of artifacts, and outline the head's contour. Manual identification of lesion and radiosensitive structures and selection of collimator diameter allow volume rendering and three-dimensional dosimetry

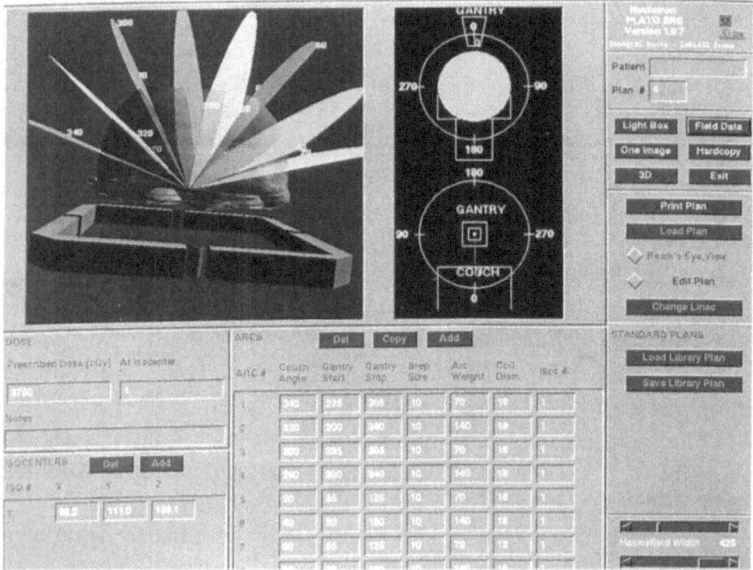

Fig. 3. Treatment planning tool. Standard nine-arc library is modified here to avoid the 360 arc at eye level

The isocenter is interactively determined: initially it is automatically located according to the lesion's geometry, then a sphere is displayed whose diameter corresponds to the chosen collimator. Covering the entire volume of the lesion with the transparent sphere represents the reference isodose (normally 80%): the three-dimensional display gives the immediate perception of this coverage.

The monitor units are calculated for each arc, according to the skin-isocenter distance. CT or MRI data can be reformatted along each of the chosen treatment arcs, in order to evaluate the anatomical structures encountered.

Based on the chosen treatment geometry and according to the physical data of the collimators and accelerator, the system calculates the dose distribution. The result can be displayed as a set of isodose curves superimposed on the original or reformatted CT and MRI images (Fig. 4). Alternatively, the isodoses can be displayed as transparent three-dimensional surfaces that are superimposed on the three-dimensional reconstruction of the lesion and of other structures of interest (optic chiasm and nerves, hypothalamus, brainstem etc). Treatment evaluation can alternatively be obtained from the volume histogram that graphically represents the percentage of the lesion volume covered by different dose values (Fig. 5).

Upon acceptance of the planned treatment, a dosimetric report is printed. This document shows all LINAC calibration data, the collimator in use, the position of isocenter, the angular values of couch and gantry, and the moni-

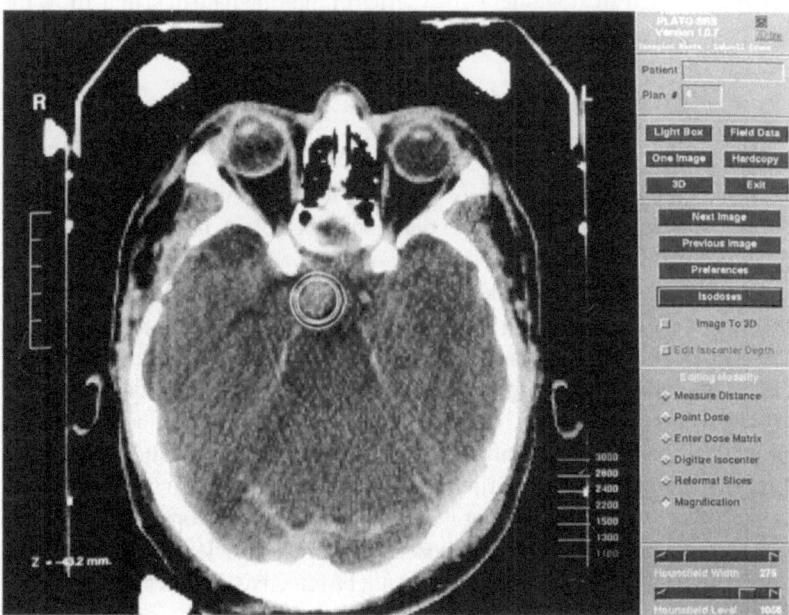

Fig. 4. Color-coded isodose curves displayed on original CT slice

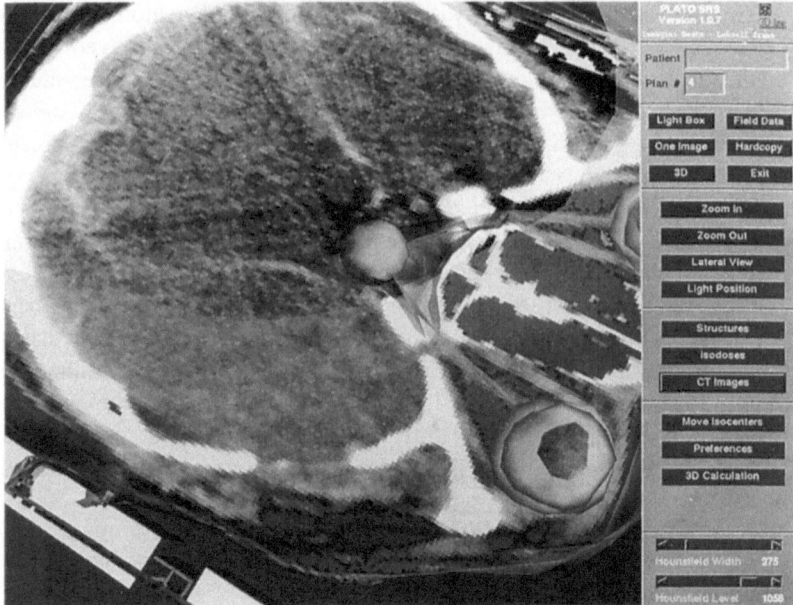

Fig. 5. Isodose transparent volume, wrapping the lesion; here a 2200-cGy dose

tor units of each arc, together with a series of intermediate data that allow the physicist to evaluate the procedure.

Discussion

In spite of their benign histology and well-defined limits with respect to the surrounding healthy parenchyma, conditions that seem to be ideal for radiosurgical treatment, reports on the outcome of this therapeutic approach on craniopharyngiomas are scarce. The availability of high anatomical definition using contemporary neuroimaging modalities will certainly increase the interest for this therapeutic choice: MRI imaging technique, with the display of coronal and sagittal planes showing the position of optic nerves and chiasm, will increase the precision with which the tumor borders can be outlined. Three-dimensional dose planning software, already available for Gamma Units and LINACS, allows precise description of isodose distribution. At the same time it is likely that, with the increasing imitations established for optic nerve irradiation (reported maximal tolerated dose on the order of 8-10 Gy), the maximal dose delivered at the tumor border may not be effective, even with an extremely steep dose drop off.

For this reason we believe that an effective radiotherapeutic approach can only be achieved using a fractionated stereotactic approach and a repositiona-

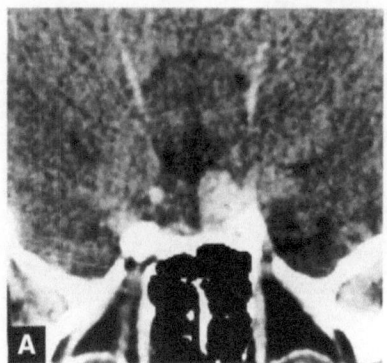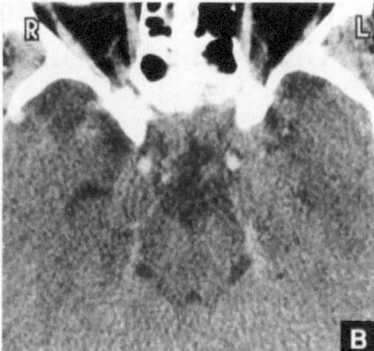

Fig. 6. A Postoperative craniopharyngioma recurrence after 1 year; **B** 6-month follow-up after stereotactic LINAC boost (2200 cGy), followed by stereotactic fractionated further treatment (200 cGy in 13 sessions). No visual worsening has been recorded

ble localizer, whose effect could be completed, if necessary, by a radiosurgical "boost." This approach will benefit from the advantage of localization, offered by the stereotactic tecnique combined with the lower radiotoxicity guaranteed by the fractionated treatment on surrounding delicate structures (Fig. 6 a, b).

References

Backlund EO, Rahn T, Sarby B, deSchryver A, Wennerstrand J (1972a) Closed stereotactic hypophysectomy by means of 69 Co Gamma radiation. Acta Radiol 13:368-376

Backlund EO, Johannson L, Sarby B (1972b) Studies on craniopharyngiomas. II. Treatment by stereotactic radiosurgery. Acta Chir Scand 138:749-759

Betti OO, Munari C, Rosler R (1989) Stereotactic radiosurgery with the linear accelerator. Treatment of arteriovenous malformations. Neurosurgery 24:311-321

Colombo F, Benedetti A, Pozza F, Avanzo RC, Marchetti C, Chierego G, Zanardo A (1985) External stereotactic irradiation by linear accelerator. Neurosurgery 16:154-160

Kjellberg GH, Hanamura T, Davis KR, Lyons S, Butler W, Adams R (1983) Bragg peak proton beam therapy for arteriovenous malformations of the brain. N Engl J Med 309:269-274

Leksell L (1951) The stereotactic method and radiosurgery of the brain. Acta Chir Scand 102:316-319

Leksell L (1983) Stereotactic radiosurgery. J Neurosurg Psychiatry 46:797-803

Noren G, Arndt J, Hindmarsh T (1983) Stereotactic radiosurgery in cases of acoustic neurinoma: further experiences. Neurosurgery 13:12-22

Steiner L, Lindquist CH (1987) Radiosurgery in cerebral arteriovenous malformations. In: Taskar RR (ed) Stereotactic surgery. Hanley and Belfus, Philadelphia, pp 329-336 (Neurosurgery: state of the arts reviews)

Endocrine Tests and Hormonal Therapy in Craniopharyngioma

R. Cozzi, G. Oppizzi, P. Orlandi, D. Dallabonzana, and I. Chiodini

Introduction

The hypothalamus exerts control over the anterior pituitary gland and synthesizes hormones of the posterior pituitary: vasopressin and oxytocin are synthesized in the hypothalamic-supraoptic and paraventricular nuclei: they migrate along neuronal axons of the supraoptic-pituitary tract and terminate in the posterior pituitary where they are stored and released into the systemic circulation. Hypothalamic control of anterior pituitary secretion is exerted by neurotransmitters and neurohormones that reach the pituitary by the hypothalamo-pituitary portal system and stimulate or inhibit the secretion of pituitary hormones (Table 1).

In patients with craniopharyngioma, endocrine symptoms are explained by a deficiency in hypophysiotropic hormone secretion and/or by the occurrence of a hypothalamic-pituitary disconnection due to the compression of the pituitary stalk by the tumor. The initial symptoms in children and adolescents are predominantly endocrinologic; however, these manifestations frequently go unrecognized and at diagnosis over 80% of patients have hypothalamic pituitary endocrine deficiencies (Jenkins et al. 1976). These endocrine abnormalities may precede the manifestation of symptoms by months or years; even in adults endocrine manifestations usually precede the late neurological manifestations (Bartlett 1971).

In prepuberal patients sexual precocity is often associated with neurological symptoms; in young adults growth deficiency may be present with hypogonadism, and diabetes insipidus may occur. In adults hypogonadism with galactorrhea and diabetes insipidus may accompany severe neurological symptoms (Table 2).

The analytical evaluation of pituitary function shows that in patients with craniopharyngioma the secretion of growth hormone (GH) and of gonadotropins (luteinizing hormone LH; follicle-stimulating hormone, FSH) is im-

Div. Endocrinology, Ospedale Niguarda, Piazza Ospedale Maggiore 3, 20162 Milan, Italy

paired in most patients; in contrast, the secretion of the other hormones is less affected (Jenkins et al. 1976; Table 3).

Clinical manifestations of hypothalamic pituitary insufficiency are generally similar to those related to primary pituitary lesions, with some excep-

Table 1. Hypothalamic hormones

Hormones	+	−	Location
Posterior pituitary hormones			
• Arginine vasopressin			Supraoptic and para-
• Oxytocin			ventricular nucleus
Hypophysyotropic hormones			
• TRH	TSH, PRL		Paraventricular nucleus
• GnRH	LH, FSH		Preoptic area
• Somatostatin		GH, TSH	Periventricular nucleus
• GHRH	GH		Arcuate nucleus
• PIH, dopamine		PRL	Arcuate nucleus
• CRH	ACTH		Paraventricular nucleus

See text for abbreviations.
+/-; stimulatory/inhibitory effect

Table 2. Age-related signs and symptoms of parasellar tumors

Age	Symptom	
Before puberty	Headache Vomiting Sexual precocity	
Young adults	Sexual infantilism	(absent or arrested puberty)
	Growth deficiency	
	Hypogonadism	(impotence, loss of libido, amenorrhea)
	Diabetes insipidus	
	Obesity	
Adults	Headache Visual disturbances Asthenia Galactorrhea Diabetes insipidus Hypogonadism	

Table 3. Hypothalamic pituitary function in patients with craniopharyngioma (from Jenkins et al. 1976)

	n	%
GH deficiency	19/20	95
Gonadotropin deficiency	19/20	95
Pituitary-adrenal dysfunction	10/20	50
Secondary hypothyroidism	13/20	65
Hyperprolactinemia	10/20	50
Diabetes insipidus	5/20	25

tions. Even basal evaluation of pituitary hormones does not distinguish between hypothalamic and pituitary origin of the lesion. Therefore in patients in whom a hypothalamic lesion is highly suspected, only a dynamic evaluation of pituitary hormones (using stimulatory neurotransmitters) may support, together with the clinical features, the findings of the neuroradiological study.

Evaluation of the Secretion of Anterior Pituitary Hormones

GH Secretion

The assessment of GH levels in a single blood sample does not have any clinical significance since GH is secreted in episodic peaks that are interspersed with periods with little or no secretion. In craniopharyngioma lower or absent spontaneous GH pulses may be present; however, the evaluation of the pattern of 24-h GH secretion requires assessment of several blood samples, a very expensive maneuver. Therefore the evaluation of GH secretion is performed by provocative tests; insulin-induced hypoglycemia (IIH), arginine, clonidine, L-dopa are the classical, most used tests for evaluation of GH secretion (Table 4). Most investigators consider responses to these stimuli to less than 7-10 ng/ml as suggestive of an impairment of GH secretion. Indeed, in patients with craniopharyngioma lower or no responses are observed. These agents exert their effect at the hypothalamic level and require a normal hypothalamic-pituitary axis. Therefore the impairment of GH response to these stimuli means that a defect in the hypothalamic-pituitary axis exists, but does not differentiate hypothalamic from pituitary disease.

In contrast, GHRH, the physiological releasing hormone of GH, directly stimulates GH-secreting cells: the administration of this agent (1 γ/kg i.v.) induces an increase of plasma GH levels, reaching peak values from 10 to 100 ng/ml after 15-30 min. In patients with primitive pituitary lesions the

Table 4. Evaluation of growth hormone (GH) secretion

Test	Test conditions	Time of GH response (min)
Insulin	Regular insulin (0.05-0.1 U/kg iv); 50% fall in blood glucose is necessary for adequate testing; nadir blood glucose levels 20-30 min after insulin	45-75
Arginine	L-Arginine (5%-10% solution; 0.5 g/kg, 30 g for adults) infused over 30 min	60-120
L-Dopa	0.5 g p.o.	120-180
Clonidine	0.15 mcg/m^2	60-120

response to this acute test is reduced or absent; in contrast, it is usually maintained in subjects with hypothalamic damage (Fig. 1). However, this distinction is not always so definite, since even in patients with craniopharyngioma the lack of GH response may occur due to the chronic endogenous GHRH deficiency (Delitala 1989).

GH secretory status is reflected even by plasma levels of somatomedin C (or insulin-like growth factor I, IGF-I), a peptide that belongs to the family of tissue growth factors; it is synthesized in multiple organs and tissues, with the highest tissue concentration and synthesis found in the liver (Van Wik 1984). IGF-I levels are stable due to its long half-life and are correlated with plasma integrated 24-h GH concentration. In patients with craniopharyngioma and GH deficiency, low levels of IGF-I (values below 0.5 U/ml) have often been found.

In children operated on for craniopharyngioma the serum IGF-I concentration may be normal in the face of GH deficiency (Bucher et al. 1983). These children (who have normal or excessive linear growth) frequently exhibit hyperphagia and excessive weight gain and sometimes have elevated prolactin (PRL) and insulin levels, which might support the linear growth.

Another index of GH secretory activity is IGFBP-3, a binding protein of IGF-I, whose levels are GH dependent. Levels are reduced in states of GH deficiency (Furlanetto 1984).

Thyroid Function

The evaluation of thyroid function in patients with craniopharyngioma quite regularly shows low or normal free-T3 and free-T4 levels, and low, normal, or slightly high basal TSH (thyroid-stimulating hormone) levels. In addition

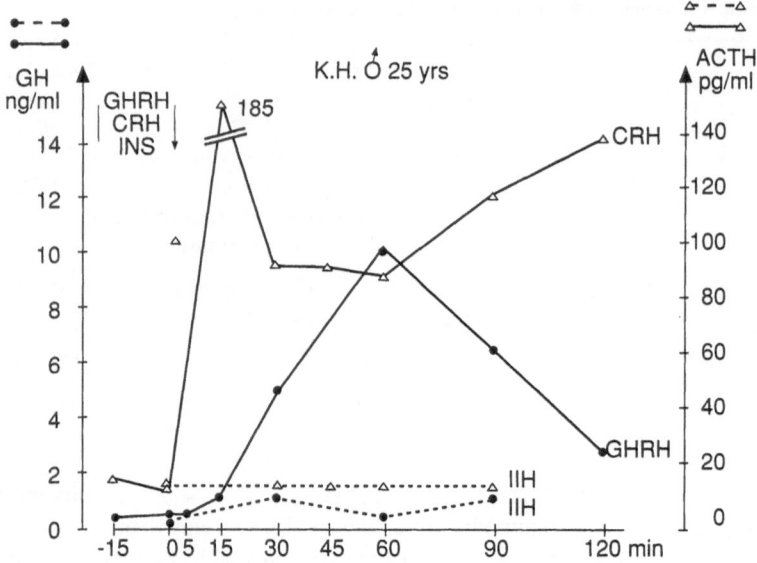

Fig. 1. Stimulation of secretion of GH (*solid circles*) and ACTH (*open triangles*) by IIH (*dashed line*) and by CRH and GHRH (*solid lines*) in a patient with craniopharyngioma

there is low biological THS activity due to an alteration of its synthesis by the pituitary. Dissociation of bioassayable from immunoassayable TSH can lead to the apparently paradoxical finding of normal or even elevated levels of TSH in hypothalamic hypothyroidism.

The administration of TRH (the releasing hormone of TSH, 200-400 γ i.v.) has been suggested to test for the anatomical site of the lesion. In hypothalamic hypothyroidism the typical pituitary response to TRH administration is an enhanced and somewhat delayed peak (attributed to an associated GH deficiency that sensitizes the pituitary to TRH), wherease the response to TRH in patients with intrinsic pituitary TSH failure is abnormal. However, in actual practice the TSH responses in hypothalamic and pituitary disease overlap substantially and do not allow the site of the lesion to be distinguished (Snyder et al. 1974).

Adrenal Function

The adrenal function is evaluated by determining urinary free cortisol (UFC) that reflects the 24-h cortisol production rate; in contrast the assessment of plasma levels of adrenocorticotropic hormone (ACTH) and cortisol in single morning blood samples is not indicative of the daily cortisol secretion pattern, since the secretion of these hormones occurs by a circadian rhythm and is related to stress. Patients with craniopharyngioma may have normal or low levels of UFC.

To evaluate the presence of hypothalamic-pituitary-hypoadrenocorticism, tests as IIH and corticotrophin-releasing hormone (CRH) administration have been proposed. IIH (0.05-0.1 U/kg i.v.), which acts at the hypothalamic level, may show low or absent responses in terms of ACTH and cortisol serum levels in both hypothalamic and pituitary lesions. In contrast, the corticotropin-releasing hormone (CRH) test (1 γ/kg i.v.) may indicate the hypothalamic origin of the lesion: indeed, whereas patients with hypothalamic pituitary-adrenal insufficiency usually have an exaggerated response, in patients with pituitary-adrenal deficiency there is little or no ACTH and cortisol response to CRH administration (Fig. 1; Muller et al. 1986).

Gonadal Function

The levels of gonadal sex hormones, testosterone, and 17β estradiol are regularly low. LH and FSH plasma levels are low and the evaluation of their pulsatility (assessed by blood samples taken at 15-min intervals for 4 h) shows the absence of the normal daily fluctuations. The acute administration of gonadotropin releasing hormone (GnRH) often does not induce any FSH and LH response either in hypothalamic lesions or in pituitary disorders. The absent or diminished pituitary response results both from lack of priming with GnRH (which in most instances depends on hypothalamic GnRH deficiency) and from the lack of sex hormone pituitary receptors. Therefore the GnRH test is considered useless both in the diagnosis of hypothalamic pituitary hypogonadism and in locating the origin of the disease (Wass and Besser 1989).

PRL Levels

An inhibitory tonic control on PRL secretion is exerted by hypothalamic dopamine, which reaches pituitary dopamine receptors via tuberoinfundibular pathways. This finding explains why increased PRL levels are observed not only in PRL-secreting pituitary adenomas, but also in those lesions impinging the pituitary stalk or in clinical disorders in which antidopaminergic drugs are used.

Since a single blood sample for PRL assessment may often show high values due to venipuncture or to stress, PRL levels have to be assessed in at least three blood samples taken at 20-min intervals. In patients with hypothalamic lesions PRL levels may even be normal (up to 25 ng/ml) or slightly increased (up to 50-70 ng/ml): the increase of PRL levels is due to the hypothalamic-pituitary disconnection caused by the tumor mass effect. In contrast, higher PRL levels (greater than 100 ng/ml) are strongly suggestive of the presence of a PRL-secreting pituitary adenoma.

Evaluation of the Secretion of Posterior Pituitary Hormones: Diabetes Insipidus

Diabetes insipidus is the most frequent disorder linked to a dysfunction of the neurohypophysis in patients with craniopharyngioma. In patients with neurological deficit, such as bitemporal hemianopsia, a polyuric state obviously points to central diabetes insipidus. In patients with complete diabetes insipidus urine osmolality does not increase over plasma osmolality in response to water deprivation but shows a greater than 50% increase in urine osmolality in response to vasopressin injection. In patients with partial diabetes insipidus the urine may become concentrated to some degree in response to water deprivation, but urine osmolality also increases by at least 10% after vasopressin injection.

Hormone Replacement Therapy

Replacement therapy must be tailored to the individual hormone deficiency and, if possible, should not be instituted until the hypothalamic-pituitary-adrenal axis has been assessed (Table 5). For example, thyroid hormone replacement before institution of glucocorticoid therapy in a cortisol-deficient subject may precipitate an adrenal crisis.

Table 5. Replacement therapy

Adrenal	Hydrocortisone acetate (25-37.5 mg/day) or prednisone (5-7.5 mg/day)
Thyroid	L-thyroxine (100 γ/day)
Gonads	
• Male	Testosterone (enanthate, 100-200 mg monthly), gonadotropins or LHRH (by pump)
• Female	Estroprogestinic hormones (pill); gonadotropins or LHRH (by pump)
Growth	Growth hormone (0.06-0.09 U/kg per day)
Diabetes insipidus	Desmopressin (DDAVP) (5-15 µg/day once-three times/day)
	⎧ Chlorpropamide (250-500 mg/day)
	⎪ Carbamazepine (400-600 mg/day), milder forms
	⎨ Clofibrate (1.0-2.0 g/day)
	⎩ Hydrochlorothiazide (50-100 mg/day)

Cortisol Deficiency

Cortisol deficiency is usually treated by oral administration of 25 mg of hydrocortisone on awakening and 12.5 mg at 4-6 p.m. This is the simplest way to simulate the circadian rhythm of cortisol secretion. Some patients require a lower dose. Alternatively, synthetic glucocorticoids may be used, either a prednisone dose of 5 mg on awakening and 2.5 mg in the afternoon or dexamethasone (0.5 + 0.25 mg). During stress - whether psychological or physical - fever, and illness, the dose is usually increased to an equivalent of 25 mg hydrocortisone every 6 to 8 h. If parenteral administration is required, 50-100 mg hydrocortisone is given every 6 h. The starting of glucocorticoid therapy can give clinical evidence of diabetes insipidus.

Thyroid Hormone Deficiency

Thyroid hormone deficiency is treated with levothyroxine; the oral dose usually ranges from 0.075 mg to 0.1 mg once daily. The dose is adjusted according to the clinical response, and the serum T3 level should be in the middle to upper part of the normal range. Measurement of serum TSH is of no value in assessing response to levothyroxine in patients with hypothalamic-pituitary disease.

Gonadal Steroids Deficiency

In man testosterone enanthate is usually administered i.m., 200 mg every 15-30 days. When initiating testosterone therapy i.m., it is advisable to begin with a low dose and gradually increase it. Adequacy of therapy is assessed by measuring serum testosterone concentrations just before the scheduled injection.

In hypogonadal women estrogen replacement therapy is given to maintain or to promote feminization and to prevent bone loss. There are numerous regimens for estrogen replacement. Estrogens are administered cyclically with appropriate progestogens; this is easily achieved by administering one of the several low-dose oral contraceptive preparations containing 30 γ ethynil-estradiol. Alternatively, estrogens can be given for 3 of 4 weeks by cutaneous patches and a small dose of progestogen administered for the last 10-12 days of estrogen treatment.

To initiate puberty and to restore fertility gonadotropins and GnRH may be given (Claman and Seibell 1990). Since the underlying defect is at the hypothalamic level, usually after short-term administration of GnRH plasma LH and FSH levels increase in about 50% of the patients; after repetitive treatment for 5 days or longer, plasma gonadotropin levels rise to the normal range in most patients with hypothalamic defect, but not in individuals with panhypopituitarism. The more severe the deficiency, the longer GnRH has to be administered to restore gonadotropin secretion. The long-term administration of LHRH in a pulsatile manner by peristaltic micropumps results in the achievement of the normal gonadal function in both sexes, normal pulsatile LH secretion, normal mean levels of plasma LH and FSH and, in most, ovulatory menses or mature sperm in the ejaculate.

Growth Hormone Substitution Therapy

In the past years the aim of treatment of GH deficiency was to promote normal growth rates in children and GH treatment was traditionally withdrawn when patients reached puberty. Recently, however, the findings showing that GH exerts important regulatory actions on metabolic homeostasis even in normal adults prompted the study of effects of GH substitution therapy in GH-deficient adults who had received GH only in childhood or not at all.

As for growth rates, in some patients operated on for craniopharyngioma a spontaneous catch-up growth phenomenon is observed after surgery and occurs even if GH secretion is impaired (see above; Fig. 2, upper panel). In contrast, for patients needing GH treatment, the growth rates increased up to 8-10 cm/year during the first 12 months of treatment with a dose of 0.05 mg (0.1 U)/kg body weight three times weekly (Fig. 2, lower panel). Nowadays, due to the unlimited availability of biosynthetic GH, substitution treatment can be performed with a dose quite similar to the amount of the daily GH secretion rate observed in normal children: because the growth response is a function of the dose given, the dose 0.05 mg (0.1 U)/kg administered daily produces a more rapid growth and no increase in the occurrence of side effects.

In children with idiopathic, isolated GH deficiency early recognition of the deficiency and early treatment are very important, since every day that a child grows at a low rate contributes to loss of ultimate stature; in contrast GH treatment works better in a child with craniopharyngioma who has grown normally before he acquires GH deficiency.

As for adults, recent reports have generated intriguing evidence for several detrimental consequences of GH deficiency in these patients. Among the most significant are the epidemiological reports of an increased prevalence of cardiovascular mortality and shortened life expectancy (Rosen and Bengtsson 1990). In addition, chronic GH deficiency induces a depressed mood, a decreased bone density, and abnormal body composition and metabolism, i.e., lean body mass and hydration state decrease, fat mass increases (Cuneo et al. 1992). These changes are reverted by GH therapy, which has been

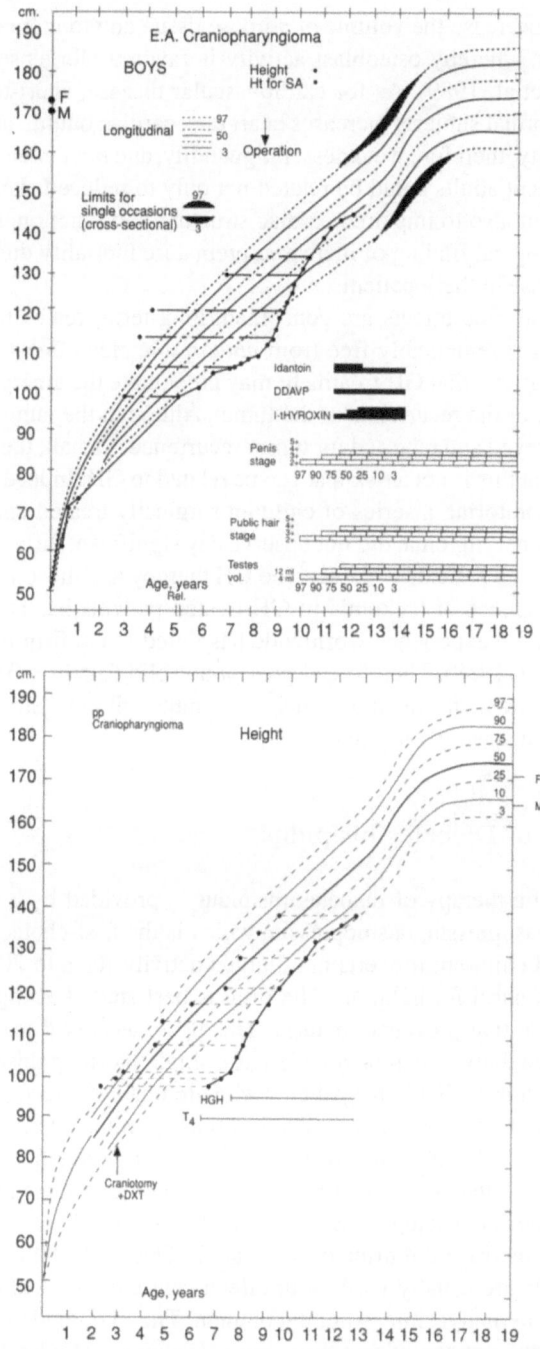

Fig. 2. Linear growth in craniopharyngioma. *Upper panel*: spontaneous catch-up growth after operation. *Lower panel*: the effect of GH treatment

shown to decrease the volume of adipose tissue and to increase the amount of muscle, whereby osteoblast activity is favored (Jorgensen et al. 1989; Salomon et al. 1989). As for cardiovascular disease, short-term GH treatment in normal subjects increases heart rate, cardiac output, and myocardial contractility; therefore weakness, fatiguability, and poor exercise capacity in GH-deficient adults could be related not only to reduced skeletal mass and strength but also to impaired cardiac structure and function, supporting the epidemiological finding of increased premature mortality due to cardiovascular disease in these patients.

As far as side effects are concerned, long-term treatment with recombinant GH is remarkably free from undesirable side effects. Nevertheless, concerns persist that GH treatment may precipitate the emergence of an occult tumor or the recurrence of the tumor. Although the number of such patients surveyed and reported for tumor recurrence is small, the data available suggest that this is not a risk that can be related to GH. Indeed, Clayton et al. (1988), monitoring a series of children surgically treated and/or irradiated for craniopharyngioma, did not observe any significant differences in recurrence between patients who received GH therapy and those who did not. An excess incidence of leukemia in GH-treated patients has been reported in Japan, but the experience worldwide has failed to confirm this association (Fisher et al. 1988). Therefore at present no solid data link GH use with the induction or enhancement of malignancy, although more studies and observation are needed in this area.

Therapy of Diabetes Insipidus

The specific therapy of diabetes insipidus is provided by a synthetic analogue of vasopressin, desmopressin, which is the first-choice drug for both adults and children; it exerts antidiuretic activity for 8 to 20 h and can be taken as a nasal formulation. The drug is best started at night to find the lowest dose that prevents nocturia. This dose, usually 5 to 10 µg, can be given twice daily or can be doubled as a single morning dose. A parenteral formulation is available for patients who are unable to take the drug by the nasal route. Desmopressin can also be effective when administered orally.

For patients having some residual vasopressin production (partial diabetes insipidus), the oral hypoglycemic agent chlorpropamide may ameliorate symptoms by enhancing the action of small amounts of vasopressin on renal tubules to increase the urine concentration. Doses of 250 to 750 mg chlorpropamide are usually used, with effectiveness in 50%-80% of these patients, but hypoglycemia is not uncommon. The hypolipidemic agent clofibrate and the anticonvulsant drug carbamazepine may also be effective in patients with partial diabetes insipidus, by directly stimulating the release of vasopressin from the hypothalamus. In addition, carbamazepine works at the renal level. Finally, thiazide diuretics (50-100 mg hydrochlotiazide daily) may reduce the volume of urine by causing mild salt depletion.

References

Bartlett JR (1971) Craniopharyngiomas: summary of 85 cases. J Neurol Neurosurg Psychiatry 34:37-41

Bucher H, Zapf J, Torresani T (1983) Insulin like growth factors I and II, prolactin and insulin in 19 growth hormone deficient children with excessive, normal or decreased longitudinal growth after operation for craniopharyngioma. New Engl J Med 309:1142-1146

Claman P, Seibell MM (1990) Ovulation induction: GnRH. In: Seibell MM (ed) Infertility. Appleton and Lange, Norwalk, pp 333-350

Clayton PE, Price DA, Shalet SM, Gattemaneni HR (1988) Craniopharyngioma recurrence and growth hormone therapy. Lancet 1:642

Cuneo RC, Salomon F, Mc Gauley GA, Sonksen PH (1992) The growth hormone deficiency syndrome in adults. Clin Endocrinol 37:387-397

Delitala G (1989) Clinical neuropharmacology in the management of disorders of the pituitary and hypothalamus. In: De Groot LJ et al (eds) Endocrinology, 2nd edn. Saunders, Philadelphia, pp 454-473

Fisher DA, Job JC, Preece M (1988) Growth hormone deficiency, human growth hormone and the occurrence of leukemia. Lancet 1:1159-1160

Furlanetto RW (1984) Plasma forms of somatomedin and the binding protein phenomenon. Clin Endocrinol Metab 13:31-42

Jenkins JS, Gilbert CJ, Ang V (1976) Hypothalamic-pituitary function in patients with craniopharyngiomas. J Clin Endocrinol Metab 43:394-399

Jorgensen JOL, Pedersen SA, Thuesen LT (1989) Beneficial effects of growth hormone treatment in GH-deficient adults. Lancet ii:1221-1224

Muller OA, Schopol J, Stalla GH, Stalla J, von Werder K (1986) CRF in the diagnosis of disorders of the hypothalamo-pituitary-adrenal system. In: Muller EE, Mc Leod RM (eds) Neuroendocrine perspectives, vol 5. Elsevier, Amsterdam, pp 73-85

Rosen T, Bengtsson BA (1990) Premature cardiovascular mortality in hypopituitarism-a study of 333 consecutive patients. Lancet 336:285-289

Salomon F, Cuneo RC, Hesp R, Sonksen PH (1989) The effects of treatment with recombinant human growth hormone on body composition and metabolism in adults with growth hormone deficiency. New Engl J Med 26:1797-1803

Snyder PJ, Jacobs LS, Rabello MM, Sterling FM, Shore RN, Utiger ND, Daughaday WH (1974) Diagnostic value of thyrotropin-releasing hormone in pituitary and hypothalamic diseases: assessment of thyrotropin and prolactin secretion in 100 patients. Ann Intern Med 81:751-757

Van Wik JJ (1984) The somatomedins: biologic actions and physiologic control mechanisms. In: Li CH (ed) Hormonal proteins and peptides, vol 12. Academic, New York, pp 81-125

Wass J, Besser GM (1989) Tests of pituitary function. In: De Groot LJ et al (eds) Endocrinology, 2nd edn, Saunders, Philadelphia, pp 492-502

Concluding Remarks

G. Broggi, Editor

All the material in this book, and, in particular, the preceding chapters deal with the findings presented by various authors at the workshop "Craniopharyngiomas: Surgical Treatment" held in Milan, Italy, on May 14, 1993. The editor considers it worthwhile the reader to append the transcription of the round table discussion and the following comments put forth at this workshop.

The round table was chaired by Giovanni Broggi, who divided the discussion into five main topics. The first topic was pituitary-diencephalic disturbances, the second neuropsychological disturbances, the third different surgical approaches, the fourth the problem of recurrence, and finally the training of neurosurgeons who want to approach the surgery of craniopharyngiomas.

The round table was opened by Broggi, recalling a discussion on the clinical abnormalities induced by the presence of craniopharyngiomas that are mainly due to an alteration of the hypothalamic functions. In this regard it must be said that there are differences between children and adults and, as Villani said, the major problem is the possibility of avoiding other abnormalities (apart from diabetes insipidus) by preserving the pituitary stalk in so far as possible during surgery.

Lapras showed some slides, confirming that the deficiency in growth hormone secretion and the deficiency of other hormones such as LH, DH, and FSH is completely restored to normal after surgery, as described in the literature.

Furthermore, diabetes insipidus is found in some 50% of his patients after surgery, being of three kinds: immediate that remains permanent, and this is the prevalent form; immediate and regressive is rare; and the form of diabetes insipidus whose onset is some 2 weeks after removal of craniopharyngioma.

Only 5.6% of patients operated for craniopharyngioma are completely normal from an endocrine point of view after the removal of the lesion. Death due to endocrine abnormalities induced by surgery remains important, as mentioned in the literature. Obesity after surgery may be due to an endocrine abnormality with the onset of hyperphagia; this is the cause of main neuropsychological problem patients have after surgery.

Broggi: Do you think that the preservation of the pituitary stalk during surgery can avoid the endocrine abnormalities that appear in patients, apart from diabetes insipidus? I think that it is important to discuss which approach can preserve the diencephalon best.

Carmel: I have experience on 11 patients out of 99 in whom the pituitary stalk has been preserved. These patients initially had diabetes insipidus and six of these 11 lost the requirements for DDAVP during the first 2 weeks after surgery. I think that the preservation of the stalk does not mean that the patients are pituitary normal anyhow; in fact, two of these 11 patients are under total endocrine treatment although the stalk appeared anatomically on MRI.

Lapras: According to the experience I have on 11 cases I want to add that there is the need to advise the parents of patients that pregnancy will be very difficult in the patient's future if surgery of the pituitary stalk has been made as an endocrine imbalance occurred. The other major problem related to the conditions of these patients after surgery is due to the fact that there is a consequent abnormality of thyroid function that has to be treated with thyroxine to avoid obesity. This treatment can be of psychological help to the patients. A deficency in other hormones such as growth hormone, LH, DH and FSH is completely restored after surgery, as described in the literature. Of the three kinds of diabetes insipidus that are found in 54% of the patients after surgery the most frequent form is diabetes insipidus with immediate onset that tends to remain permanent. The other two forms, the immediate and regressive and the diabetes insipidus with onset about 2 weeks after removal of craniopharyngioma, are rare. Only 5.6% of patients are completely normal endocrinologically after the removal of the craniopharyngioma. Moreover, it must be stated that mortality due to endocrine abnormalities after surgery remains important, as mentioned in the literature. Obesity after surgery may be due to an endocrine abnormality with the onset of hyperphagia and this is the major problem.

Rahn: I just want to say a few words about the last question on obesity. In our experience the behavior of hyperphagia is similar to the behavior of visual defect, because when we evacuate the cyst of the craniopharyngioma we can restore visual loss and patients stop eating too much. Moreover, some of these patients in whom the medial nuclei of the third ventricle are compressed by the cyst of the craniopharyngioma and the circulation in the nuclei is bad don't have the feeling of satisfaction and are always hungry.

Broggi: I would like to ask Rahn about his experience at Karolinska with endocrine abnormalities in patients who have been treated with gamma-knife surgery. This is a major problem that has been debated among neurosurgeons, neurologists, and pediatricians, because this morning all speakers stated that when one decides to operate on a craniopharyngioma he must be radical and even if may induce some abnormalities of the endocrine system.

Rahn: When patients develop an endocrine abnormality, of which the most frequent is a GH deficiency, they usually continue to have that deficiency even after surgery and these already preoperatively deficient patients account for about 85% of all patients in our series.

Scannavini: As the diencephalic syndrome after surgery is very important and very severe, what are the real risks of manipulation of the hypothalamic structures in the removal of the craniopharyngioma?

Lapras: This is a problem related to the surgical technique we use.

Carmel: Just to remind you that to have hypothalamic abnormalities you need to have bilateral hypothalamic damage. In surgery the problem is another and it is related to the fact that the tumor is lodged in original hypothalamic structures that, once the tumor is removed, keeping the arachnoid plane of the tumor intact, you restore all the hypothalamic structures, and so you may have normal hypothalamic function after surgery. Moreover, after surgery you observe the excursion of many centimeters of the hypothalamic structures without any deficit, contrary to the fact that if you stretch the cranial nerve during surgery you induce a deficit.

Lapras: I totally agree with you.

Fraioli: Three questions: the first: do you consider a solid craniopharyngioma, intrasellar and suprasellar reaching the lower part of the third ventricle, as an indication for transphenoidal surgery? Second question is: in the first postoperative period, is CT scan or MRI better to check the result of surgery? The third question: how do you close the cerebrospinal fluid fistula?

Nicola: The indication for the transphenoidal route, in case of solid tumor, is only in intrasellar infradiaphragmatic lesions. Occasionally a craniopharyngioma with suprasellar extension can be completely removed by a TSN approach, but, while pulling the tumor down, there is no control of the suprasellar vascular and nervous structures and, moreover, you can never be sure to obtain a real radical removal of the tumor and its capsule. As far as the third question is concerned, the best is the use of muscular tissue and to complete the closure of the sella floor with a piece of the cartilagineum septum blocked by glue.

Villani: I agree with you.

Savoiardo: In the diagnosis of craniopharyngiomas, MRI is generally superior to CT; the only exception is given by the inferior ability of MRI in recognizing calcifications which are often of great diagnostic importance. After surgery, MRI is again superior to CT in demonstrating residual tumor or other complications; however, occasionally a tiny calcified residual tumor may be easily demonstrated by CT and missed by MRI. You must also be aware of a few aspects of postcontrast studies in the postoperative period that were clearly demonstrated in a few series of operations for various lesions, including mesial temporal sclerosis, in which no postcontrast enhancement is present. The reactive tissue or "glial scar" along the margins of the operative cavity become visible as a disruption of the blood-brain barrier (and therefore as a line of postcontrast enhancement) only 4-5 days after surgery. Therefore, when an enhancing tumor is removed, there is a window, up to the third or fourth postoperative day, in which complete removal may be assessed through the demonstration of absence of enhancement. If some enhancement is present in this period, it usually indicates residual tumor. But the matter is even more complicated, and one should always obtain an MRI study with and without contrast administration. In fact, an area of hyperintensity in T1-weighted images on the wall of the operative cavity visible a few days after surgery in a postcontrast study does not always mean residual enhancing tumor; it may indicate presence of blood, which should be visible, therefore, also on the MR scan obtained without contrast; blood by-products (methemoglobin) usually become hyperintense on T1-weighted images in 4 to 8 days: but in a surgical cavity that has been irrigated with hydrogen peroxide, the change into methemoglobin may be accelerated and hyperintensity in T1-weighted images may appear as early as on the first or second day. The postcontrast enhancement of a glial scar usually lasts 4 or 5 months, but occasionally may last longer. In general, however, an enhancing nodule on an MRI performed 4-5 months after surgery indicates residual tumor.

Fraioli: I have a question for Savoiardo about the possibility to distinguish the connective tissue found after radiotherapy by possible tumor remnants or recurrence.

Savoiardo: It is often difficult to distinguish, in an irregularly enhancing tumor, partly removed and irradiated, what is the tumor and what are the postradiation changes. A careful comparison of the whole series of pre- and postoperative MR scans and detailed knowledge of the description of the operation are always necessary. Often, only follow-up studies can clarify the matter; a regressing enhancement and a shrinking mass may indicate postradiation changes, while a persistent enhancement of a growing mass indicates tumor tissue.

Broggi: Two problems I want to discuss now are related to the choice of radiosurgery versus other procedures and the use of colloids that, according to some surgeons, makes open surgery more difficult. Another problem is the use of bleomycin.

Choux: I want to ask Dr. Giorgi his opinion about the bleomycin therapy.

Giorgi: If you don't inject bleomycin into the cavity of craniopharyngioma that is in communication with the CFS space you don't have any problem. But I think that is often only a palliative treatment: in fact we notice that in some of our cases the cyst had to be evacuated again after 1, $1^{1}/_{2}$ years.

Choux: There are two different standpoints in the literature. The first one is that of many Japanese centers where bleomycin is used only in case of cystic recurrence. The other standpoint is, for example, that of Lapras who uses bleomycin before surgery. Is it true? Do you always operate the patients with bleomycin or do you now prefer to wait. The third standpoint is what we actually do in young patients without endocrine deficits: we inject bleomycin and we wait.

Lapras: My experience is only on six patients treated with bleomycin. I want to state two points: bleomycin has a fibrotic effect and we have to consider that and, as histological study has shown, bleomycin cannot cure the wall of the cyst entirely. And this is the main fact and the reason why we use bleomycin or we use it for recurrence when we don't want to perform surgery, we can repeat bleomycin after 6 months or 1 or 2 years because we let the catheter inside. The efficacy is mainly for fresh craniopharyngiomas or craniopharyngiomas in which the cystic part is prominent. With bleomycin the capsule is more resistant and so it is less prone to be broken. I think bleomycin should be used pre-operatively not as a treatment but as a preparation for surgery.

Rahn: I want to emphasize the difference between intracystic treatment with bleomycin and 90-yttrium colloid isotope treatment. The isotopic treatment is a single treatment; you just have to inject the colloid isotope with the activity according to the volume of the cyst. The short-range β irradiation will only penetrate about 0.5 mm of the cyst wall, but this is sufficient to destroy the one layer cubic cells that produce the cystic fluid.

Carmel: I have a question for Dr. Rahn. Is there any difference between the use of [^{32}P] and yttrium in the handling of a cyst, because my experience with [^{32}P] is on three patients who all had recurrences of the cyst after [^{32}P] treatment.

Rahn: I think you refer to [^{32}P] as a chromium phosphate. We used the bismuth phosphate before we started to use yttrium, which was the first isotope Leksell and Backlund started to use, and there was quite a good effect. There is a small difference in range and half-life between these two molecules. Yttrium is a little weaker in radiation and if you have the optic nerves very close to the cyst, it may be of benefit. We are satisfied with the dose we give, that is, 20.000 rads (200 Gy pure β emitted to the inside of the cyst wall). There are very few exceptional cases with recurrence.

Dolenc: How many patients did you treat with yttrium or otherwise, or, better, how many patients were admitted to a neurosurgical department for surgery after that kind of treatment? We don't have any information about that. My experience is that surgery after this treatment is very difficult. My personal experience in four cases operated on after yttrium therapy was negative in terms of a worsening of the deficit of the first cranial nerves. In this regard I have the following question: is this deficit a contraindication for surgery after yttrium therapy? I have another comment on the fact that it is true that a cyst in which the drop was instilled won't grow further and is reduced, but what happens to other cysts? We need more experience.

Broggi: This comment is very important because I think that when we decide to begin using radioactive colloids or radiosurgery for the therapy of craniopharyngioma in these patients, this treatment should be continued for long time and not immediately followed by surgery. Is it true for everyone?

Lapras: For me it is true, although I only have little experience, only two cases.

Villani: It is definitely true, although I would always try secondary surgery in symptomatic tumor regrowth, followed by external

	radiotherapy for tumor remnants. Total tumor removal is still possible, although more difficult.
Rahn:	I agree that conventional radiotherapy may induce adhesions that make surgery difficult, while I have not seen that with yttrium or gamma-knife surgery.
Broggi:	In this regard what was reported last month in Boston at the AANS Congress about stereotactic radiotherapy made with the stereotactic frame to avoid this damage is very important.
Carmel:	In my experience, surgery was not difficult after radiotherapy. After gamma-knife surgery the tumor becomes a dead mass, although there is often cystic degeneration that can worsen the clinical picture.
Rahn:	If you use a lower dose, you may induce a slow degeneration of tumor, and, remember, cystic degeneration can be evacuated by stereotactic puncture. The other advantage of gamma-knife surgery is that a child goes to the hospital just once to undergo the treatment and not daily for 4-5 weeks as in conventional radiotherapy. With gamma-knife surgery you avoid the formation of adherences around the tumor and damage of the surrounding tissue that might appear after conventional radiotherapy.
Choux:	When you decide to use radiotherapy for treatment of recurrence, is there any contraindication, when you don't see the optic pathways?
Rahn:	As gamma-knife surgery is a kind of surgery that, when applied on the optic nerve will injure it, you need a very clear MRI image to avoid them.
Dolenc:	Do you agree that gamma-knife surgery is effective in the treatment of AVM seated deep in the brain? What is the pathophysiology of this effect? Is it the effect on small vessels? With that treatment can we avoid all the perforating arteries of the supra-and parasellar region?
Rahn:	The irradiation causes a thickening of the intima in the pathological vessel. It has been observed that the size of the lumen of the pathological vessel decreases and then the vessels are obliterated completely. The normal vessel to an AVM, however, are not affected because they are structured differently. Vessels inside the pituitary may be damaged and undergo hyalinization after gamma-knife surgery. The risk of operating on craniopharyngiomas with gamma-knife surgery, as far as the perforating vessels to the optic nerve are concerned, is that they could be obliterated by gamma-knife surgery. I mean those going through the tumor into the optic nerve. Maybe throm-

bosis is one explanation why in one patient, during 72 h, 9 months after isotope treatment, deterioration of vision of left eye developed rapidly. This event could be caused by the obliteration of the feeding vessels from the cyst capsule. It seems to be a vascular complication because it appeared just within a few days and then stayed stable and did not improve or deteriorate.

Broggi: Let us now talk about the problem of recurrences. It seems certain that recurrences may be immediate or late within the first year, and that recurrences may be dependent on the type of craniopharyngioma we are observing.

Lapras: We suggest that radiation therapy should be used as the treatment of recurrences after the first surgical treatment. And now we are showing 16 patients with recurrences after a so-called total removal. All the patients were reoperated, and we suggest that after radiotherapy patients should not be reoperated. In five cases we were able to remove the tumor completely at second surgery, while in six patients we had only partial removal after second surgery. In some cases we had difficulties in operating after radiation therapy.

Nicola: I think that the question is whether the cystic recurrences that are mentioned are considered recurrent cystic craniopharyngioma or a collection of CSF fluid after treatment. In our series of 92 cases, the recurrence rate in children has been very high: 25%, but there are two cases of cystic recurrence which were detected at a routine follow-up CT scan and did not provoke any new symptom. These two children have not been reoperated on and are followed-up with repeated MRI. These cysts are not growing so I think that they are not true recurrences and that the decision to reoperate (we favor reoperation as treatment of recurrences) cannot be based on radiological grounds only.

Lapras: I think it is very difficult to say if it is a tumor or an arachnoid adherence.

Villani: As far as is reported in the literature a time of 2 or 3 years after surgery seems to be crucial for the recurrence of the tumor.

Lapras: In our experience, it is very difficult to have recurrences after 3 years. We operated all the recurrences and we do not apply any radiation therapy. In our cases second surgery does not seem to be more complicated than the first; in some cases it is even simpler. Moreover, if you have in young patients endocrine deficit after the first operation, after the second there is a complete endocrine deficiency. Although we do not perform any radiation therapy in our department, the cases we received from outside in whom radiation therapy was applied had a consistent number of recurrences, but we do not know if radiation therapy was applied correctly or not.

Broggi: I have one question for the audience: do you agree that the two forms of craniopharyngiomas, the first in children and the second in adults, are two neuropathologically different entities and so maybe the treatment must be different?

Lapras: I completely agree. In fact we don't use radiotherapy in children, but we use it in adults.

Carmel: I think that is very difficult to biologically distinguish a pediatric and an adult form of craniopahryngioma. My question is: is the more frequent recurrence of this tumor in children related to the exogenous growth hormones that have been used in these patients?

Choux: That is true, but now we prefer to give growth hormone to decrease obesity and to let children grow. There is no evidence and no explanation for the fact that the growth hormone can increase the growth of tumor or the recurrence.

Giombini: We definitely choose to reoperate the recurrences without any other palliative treatment, although we had some deaths, such as in two of the four cases which were due maybe to the major difficulties in operating patients that underwent radiotherapy for recurrences. Moreover, regarding the differences between tumors in children and in adults and the risk of recurrences we analyzed the Labeling index of these two populations and didn't find any significant difference between the two that would justify histological difference.

Cozzi: There are no definite data on the influence of GH therapy in inducing easier growth of the tumor nor data on the possible mechanism through which GH therapy can induce a higher incidence of leukemia.

Broggi: Let us now discuss the possibility that some remnants of the tumor may be due to a wrong surgical approach to the tumor and so perhaps we should use another surgical approach.

Carmel and Villani: We agree about the importance of the side of surgical approach and that you induce more damage with an ipsilateral approach.

Broggi: I would like now to raise the problem of the training of surgeons.

Carmel: Your question is written in a report of 2 months ago in a British neurosurgical journal about the experience in Manchester on 154 patients that were operated over 30 years coming from many centers and it appears that one surgeon operated one case every 6 years and the results are much more inferior than in the other series. The problem is then how do you recognize a good craniopharyngioma surgeon?

Konovalov: I think that not only is it important to train surgeons to operate on craniopharyngiomas but also neuroradiologists and physicians and intensive care units who encounter this type of tumor.

Villani: I agree completely with Konovalov. I think that as far as the training of neurosurgeons is concerned, we must be ready to train neurosurgeons to operate on every pathology and then he is free to choose how to further specialize, maybe in the surgery of craniopahryngioma.

Subject Index